Intermittent Fasting for Women Over 50

The Complete Guide for Beginners to Lose Weight, Detox your Body, and Promote Longevity

**© Copyright 2020 by Maggie Ramsey
All rights reserved.**

This document is geared towards providing exact and reliable information about the topic and issue covered. The publication sold with the idea that the publisher is not required to render accounting, officially permitted, or otherwise qualified services. If advice is necessary, legal or professional, a practiced individual in the profession should be ordered.

- Based on the Declaration of Principles, which was accepted and approved equally by a Committee of the American Bar Association and a Committee of Publishers and Associations.

In no way is it legal to reproduce, duplicate, or transmit any part of this document in either electronic means or printed format. Recording of this publication is strictly prohibited, and any storage of this document is not allowed unless with written permission from the publisher. All rights reserved.

The information provided herein stated to be truthful and consistent, in that any liability, in terms of inattention or otherwise, by any usage or abuse of any policies, processes, or directions contained within is the sole and utter responsibility of the recipient reader. Under no circumstances will any legal obligation or blame be held against the publisher for any reparation, damages, or monetary loss due to the information herein, either directly or indirectly.

Respective authors own all copyrights not held by the publisher.

The information herein is offered for informational purposes solely and is universal as so. The presentation of the data is without a contract or any type of guarantee assurance.

The trademarks used are without any consent, and the publication of the trademark is without permission or backing by the trademark owner. All trademarks and brands within this book are for clarifying purposes only and is a property of the owners themselves, not affiliated with this document.

Table of Contents

Introduction -- 6

History of Intermittent fasting ---------------------------- 10

What is Intermittent Fasting? ----------------------------- 14

What are the beneficial effects of intermittent fasting? -- 20

The intermittent fasting and women -------------------- 26

Advantages of Intermittent Fasting for Women ------- 29

Health tips on intermittent fasting for losing weight. 34

Intermittent Fasting step by step ------------------------- 37

The Best Food And Drinks For Intermittent Fast------ 40

Healthy Exercise to support Intermittent Fasting ---- 49

Healthy Recipes For Intermittent Fasting -------------- 54

Intermittent Fast And Keto: Should You Combine The Two? --- 58

What are the after effects of intermittent fasting? ---- 83

Intermittent fasting most suitable for women, why? 97

Intermittent fasting benefits for women --------------- 111

Tips and tricks in Intermittent Fasting ----------------- 116

Intermittent Fasting Explanatory Guide ---------------- 118

Best meals to eat during Intermittent Fasting routine
--- 139

Work out during Intermittent Fasting ------------------ 198

Descriptive Recipes For Intermittent Fasting --------- 205

Keto and Intermittent Fasting ----------------------------- 241

FAQs -- 245

Conclusion -- 255

Introduction

If you are tired of too slow, too complicated, not always useful, and which regimes cheer you up? Intermittent Fasting or periodic fasting will make you lose weight and gain health if you practice it with common sense. We tell you everything.

The intermittent fasting isn't a diet but a new way to organize the timing of your food intake (meals) to get the maximum benefits. Individually, you do not change it that you eat but when you eat it.

Intermittent fasting involves fasting for long hours (more than 12 hours), which is often like staying overnight and skipping breakfast, and then concentrating all meals of the day during a reduced time window (for example between 12 p.m. and 8 p.m.). It only concerns food, but not drinks (don't panic, you can drink your coffee!).

Why does an intermittent diet seem like a good idea for anyone interested in losing weight, but they may want to know? Is intermittent intervention effective for the heart? There was one other key aspect of intermittent fasting can help to think of this to start a new trend. The intimate fasting also is known as almost always well, but even if some of these in them.

American Journal of Clinical Nutrition conducted a relatively recent study that saw 16 men present and won a 10-week bout. In the following days, experts will consume approximately 25% of their needs previously estimated. The best has left several consultations but did not give us an oriented guide to follow. As expected, the reasons for this experiment, at least, but what remains quite interesting was what he said. The gasps were quite bright after times of only ten, but they have shown improvements in cholesterol,

LDL-chosen, very useful, and also good pressure. What made this an exciting discovery was the fact that most people had to lose more than these study studies before seeing the same ideas. It was a fascinating discovery, which stimulated a significant number of people who started trying.

The intimate fasting for those who have some beneficial effects. What makes it extremely important for anyone trying to lose weight is that women have much higher relationships with each other. When you try to lose weight, it burns a lot even after six weeks, and then it starts to burn. For those who have managed to make a proper diet and exercise, you may be struggling with a little effort, but the fast is one right solution for this.

Increasingly popular in recent years for weight loss, intermittent fasting is a food mode which consists of eating nothing for 12 hours. Ideally, by extending the fast overnight, for example, by having breakfast as late as possible or by stop eating after 6 p.m. Proponents of this method praise its quick results while the more skeptical point to its potential side effects. We take stock.

This book aims at giving guidance of intermittent fasting mainly for women. You will get started with it from the history with scientific proof, to intermittent fasting, best foods, and recipes, tips, and tricks on how to achieve your women desire weight and live a fulfilled life.

History of Intermittent fasting

When you feel the need of losing your weight and cutting down your calories you will find intermittent fasting the best way for sure. There are many ways by which you can reduce weight but intermittent fasting or periodic fasting have many benefits apart from weight loss. Eating healthy, cutting down calories that are eating in a caloric deficit, and doing workout will help you in reducing weight. Here comes the question of how the idea of intermittent fasting came into being and who discovered it?

Fasting is an ancient ritual, which has been followed over the centuries by many cultures and religions. It is important to understand that fasting and starvation are two different things and shouldn't be mixed up. Starvation is a term used when the person has no idea about the availability of the meal and there is a shortage of resources while fasting is avoiding the meals intentionally and the food is available.

Periodic fasting was used not just to cure the illnesses in ancient Egypt, Greece but also to prevent many diseases. Intermittent fasting was highly common in the Middle Ages as people sought to enjoy its benefits. It was seen that intermittent fasting not only helps in reducing weight but it also decreases insulin resistance. It is also used for the prevention of many diseases.

Intermittent fasting is the most common debate these days and so scientists are busy collecting data regarding intermittent fasting. Studies conducted by Harvard have stated that fasting improves health and those who practice intermittent fasting there are chances of increased life expectancy. This is quite obvious healthy individuals will survive longer because they will be physically active and their body will be in the best state of health.

Intermittent fasting is both physical and religiously related. Many people practice intermittent fasting as part of their religion. Like Muslims they fast in the holy month of Ramadan, Hindus observes different types of fasting according to their religion. Judaism and has several common behaviors that include Yom Kippur, the truth of some. Fasting was also observed during the political times by a very famous leader Mahatma Gandhi at the time of independence of India.

Apart from controlling blood sugar, eating just one meal one day brings more several benefits – reducing size waist, increasing muscle through increased HGH hormone assuming that the individual does not meal void of proteins, reduced blood pressure, improved lipid profile through lower LDL / Shoot, and higher HDL, reduced CRP or inflation, sound, even earlier, more significant with time as in any case, and so on.

The concept of intermittent fasting has evolved with time. Starting from the point where it was considered as starvation or due to insufficient sources people used to stay hungry for a longer period and then the term fasting was identified. From a period of fasting for hours or eating only one meal, the definition of intermittent fasting has been changed. There are many types of intermittent fasting which will be discussed in the next chapter.

What is Intermittent Fasting?

Intermittent fasting is a method of eating in which you switch between eating and fasting times. This form of fasting is not about what to eat but it explains when to eat. It includes many types like restricting the number of calories, dividing the mealtime, splitting time into hours, days, or weeks, and deciding the fasting. Every day, most people are already "fast," while sleeping. Intermittent fasting can be as easy as continuing the fast a little longer. Miss breakfast, eat your first meal at noon, and your last meal at 8 pm. Then you are fasting every day for 16 hours, theoretically speaking, and limiting your eating to an eating window of 8 hours. This is the most common type of intermittent fasting, called the process 16/8.

Individuals who practice intermittent pasting reported that they felt better and were found to be more energetic. Hunger is typically not that big of a concern, but it can be a concern at first, as the body gets used to not eating for long periods. No food is permitted during the fasting period but to keep yourself full you can have water or you can drink coffee or tea. Limited calories or low caloric food is however allowed in some forms of dieting. Intake of supplements is permitted if they have no calories.

There are many different types of this eating pattern. Every method can be effective but it depends on the individual to figure out which one works best.

The 16/8 method: This method means eating only for about 8 hours a day and fasting for about 14-16 hours. You can fit in two, three, or more meals inside the eating window.

It is quite an easy method actually because you just have to skip your breakfast and don't eat after dinner. Let's take an example. If you ate your last meal around 8 pm and you don't eat till noon the next day then you will achieve 16 hours of fasting easily. Women are seen to fast for about 14-15 hours because this much fasting period is enough for them.

The 5:2 diet: This method allows you to eat normally for 5 days a week but you have to eat only 500 to 600 calories for 2 days. It is recommended for women to eat 500 calories on the days of fasting, and for men 600. You could eat normally any day of the week, for example, except on Mondays and Thursdays. Eat 2 meals of about 250 to 300 calories. No studies are evaluating the 5:2 diet itself, as the critics rightly point out, but there is plenty of research on the effects of intermittent fasting.

Eat Stop Eat method: It requires a fast 24 hours, once or twice a week. This is a 24-hour fast that is the fasting period is from one dinner to another dinner? If you end dinner, for example, at 7 p.m. Monday and don't have dinner until 7 p.m. You completed a perfect 24 hour fast the next day. You can also keep your fasting period from breakfast to breakfast or from lunch to lunch. During the quick, water, coffee, and other zero-calorie drinks are allowed but no solid foods are allowed. To lose weight, you should keep track of the time. In other words, the same amount of food you could eat as though you hadn't been fasting at all.

Alternate-day fasting: You fast every other day, in alternate-day fasting. This system comes in many different variants. Some allow for around 500 calories during the days of fasting. Any variant of this approach has been used by several of the test-tube studies demonstrating the health benefits of intermittent fasting.

Every other day a complete fast can seem very intense, so it's not recommended for beginners. With this approach, many times a week you will go to bed very hungry, which is not very fun and is possibly unsustainable in the long run.

The Warrior Diet. This method is about consuming a heavy meal at night and eating fruits and vegetables the whole day. Basically, inside a four-hour feeding window, you're fasting all day and feasting at night. One of the first common diets to incorporate any sort of intermittent fasting was the Warrior Diet. The food options for this diet are somewhat similar to the paleo diet — mainly organic, unprocessed foods.

Spontaneous meal skipping: You don't have to pursue an intermittent fasting schedule designed to reap any of its benefits. If you don't feel like eating you can skip your meal or you can send your time in preparing or eating the food.

Some people believe that to avoid hunger or to not lose muscle mass it is necessary to eat with a gap of some hours. Your body is well prepared to tackle long stretches of starvation, let alone occasionally eating one or two meals. So, if one day you're not very hungry, miss breakfast and simply eat a balanced lunch and dinner. You can also fast when you are traveling if the food is not available. Only make sure the majority of the people are consuming nutritious foods.

Intermittent fasting works for some but not for all. Some may think that this might not be as important to women as it is to men. It is also not recommended for people who have eating disorders or are susceptible to them. If you plan to try intermittent fasting, note the consistency of the diet is important. During the eating times, you cannot binge on processed foods and hope to lose weight and improve your health.

What are the beneficial effects of intermittent fasting?

Why choose intermittent fasting? Fasting is becoming more and more popular. Over the past 30-year, numerous scientific studies have demonstrated its benefits and superiority over low-calorie diets.

Fasting improves the creation of the growth hormone required for the growth of muscles, so it is a generally excellent approach to accelerate muscle gain.

1. Enable weight loss
One of the main advantages of intermittent fasting is the potential to restore fat burning and help the pounds fall off. Intermittent fasting is preferred over many other diets because you don't need to track your calories at all and so you don't need to measure at all. IMF leads to increased burning of fat and accelerated weight loss by pushing the body to use fat stores as fuel.

Glucose is used by the body as the main source of energy after you eat food. The remaining glucose is stored by the liver and muscle in the form of glycogen. If the body will not get glucose it will use its stores to provide energy to the body because many processes going on in the body requires glucose.

When you are in a constant phase of fasting the body will use all of the glycogen and glycogen is exhausted. The body starts looking for other sources to cope up with the energy demand. Other sources include fat cells which break to provide the energy. This type of fasting is similar to a keto diet where the body is deprived of the carbohydrates and the body uses fat to fuel up the body.

2. Improves Sugar in the Blood

Glucose is the simplified form of complex carbohydrates. When the food is ingested glucose is absorbed by the body.

Insulin is released by the pancreas which transfers the glucose from the bloodstream to the cells where it can be utilized. Insulin doesn't work properly in diabetic patients and so they have high blood sugar which also causes symptoms in diabetic patients like increased thirst, hunger, and urination, etc. Intermittent fasting maintains the sugar level and prevents crashes and spikes.

3. Maintains a balanced heart

One of the most remarkable advantages of intermittent fasting is its positive impact on cardiac health. Studies indicate that intermittent fasting increases heart health by reducing certain risk factors for heart disease. A study reported the great effect of intermittent fasting on many parts of the heart. It increased healthy HDL cholesterol and decreased levels of both poor LDL and triglyceride cholesterol.

4. Reduces inflammation

Inflammation is a response to any injury acquired by the body. This response is generated by the immune system. A study found that during Ramadan fasting, individuals who fast in Ramadan had decreased levels of certain inflammatory markers. Another research showed that a longer nighttime fasting cycle was correlated with a decrease in inflammation markers. In other studies, it was found that alternate-day fasting helped to suppress oxidative stress markers.

5. Healthy for your brain

Intermittent fasting not only improves the function of the heart but it also helps the brain. Some studies reported a positive impact on the brain because it has anti-inflammatory effects that delay the development of many neurodegenerative diseases mainly Alzheimer's disease.

Some also claim that fasting encourages autophagy, or "self-eating," which is our natural cellular regeneration phase of the body — a process that is improved by fasting, but more scientific evidence is needed before this is clear.

6. Reduces hunger

Fat cells produce a hormone called leptin which tells the body to stop eating. It is a satiety hormone. Your amount of leptin decreases when you're hungry, and rises when you feel finished. Since leptin is released in the fat cells, those that are obese or overweight appear to have higher levels of leptin circulating throughout the body. But too much leptin floating around can trigger leptin resistance, making it harder to effectively toggle off hunger signals. One research assessed leptin levels during intermittent fasting and found that during the fasting time, levels were lower at night.

Ghrelin is the other hormone that regulates hunger and is secreted by the brain, stomach, and intestine. It generally emits before the meals we usually eat. It is as if it is preparing our body to digest or reminds us that it is soon time to eat. However, with fasting, ghrelin gradually decreases. So be less and less hungry before your usual meals.

The intermittent fasting and women

Females are seen as more sensitive to calorie restriction and so the effects of intermittent fasting will be different in men and women. Women are found to be more susceptible to hunger signs. When the body is in a constant state of fasting it will increase the production of the satiety hormones that is leptin and ghrelin and the body will get to know that it needs food and the person should eat by now. If the body will not get enough food or it will stay deprived of food for hours then all the mechanisms of the body will stop automatically because they need sufficient energy to work. This will also affect the hormone cycle and the procedure through which another human being is born. This is the normal manner in which the body prevents a possible pregnancy, even if you are not currently pregnant or attempting to conceive.

This is the body's defense mechanism. The body gets confused between starvation and intermittent fasting.

Is periodic fasting Safe? Know that you can only last for 12 to 16 hours, and not for days at a time. You still have plenty of time to enjoy a balanced and fulfilling diet. Some older women can need to eat regularly, due to metabolic disorders or medication instructions. In any situation, you can speak to your health care provider about your eating habits before making any adjustments.

Since all the hormones are so deeply interconnected, if one hormone is set off control, the other hormones are all adversely affected. It is like it's a chain reaction. You don't want to disrupt their daily rhythm as "messengers" who regulate much of your body's roles — from energy intake to digestion, metabolism, and blood pressure.

You may wonder, with all these disadvantages will you go for intermittent fasting as a female? If you take a more positive approach then yes is the answer. Intermittent fasting will still help you meet your weight loss goals and offer additional benefits as well, if done within a short time frame, without messing with your hormones.

Intermittent fasting for menopausal and postmenopausal women is having great results. In post-menopause research, women lose twice as much weight as premenopausal women because of poorer dietary adherence. These findings suggest that after menopause fasting can be of particular benefit to women.

Advantages of Intermittent Fasting for Women

The general benefits motivating women to take up intermittent fasting include:
- The enhanced build-up of lean muscles
- Strengthening
- Weight loss continues
- Increased stress reaction in cells
- Reduction in Inflammation and oxidative stress
- Improving insulin sensitivity in overweight women
- Improved cognitive function thanks to increased production of nerve growth factor.

The most significant and immediate advantage you will reap from the IF is weight loss. Other benefits include cell repair, better mental health, and reduced insulin resistance. How weight loss is achieved? The intake of daily meals within a shorter period leaves you feeling sated all day long.

The sensation of being fuller stops you from snacking between meals. The body goes into a fasted state during fasting. This state promotes fat burning that in the fed state had been unavailable. After the last meal, you take the body enters the fasted process in around 8-12 hours. This is why you can lose weight without adjusting the type and amount of food you consume, as well as the duration of your workouts.

With age, the metabolism slows down. While fewer calories are needed to hold the weight of women over 40 years old. Women over 40 are typically exposed to pre- and post-menopausal periods and the deposition of fat in the midsection is increased. It is difficult to lose belly fat and it is linked with many complications such as high cholesterol levels, raised blood pressure, and type II diabetes.

Intermittent fasting to prevent such problems is an excellent way to keep you fit and safe. Intermittent fasting helps in reducing belly fat and the reason is the production of human growth hormone which aids in fat loss. The levels of HGH increase when the insulin content is low. Low insulin in turn will increase the HGH and this will result in increased burning of fat. To achieve good results try to do exercise, take good sleep, and fast.

Studies have shown explicitly that the use of therapeutic fasting is of benefit to women's reproductive health. This is because in women intermittent fasting can improve multiple endocrine-related health disorders including polycystic ovarian syndrome (PCOS), obesity, and metabolic syndrome.

One research specifically conducted on women with PCOS concluded that fasting decreased levels of stress neurohormone which had a positive impact on both mental and physical health. Some studies suggested that practicing caloric restriction for a shorter period normalizes the levels of luteinizing hormone which is secreted by the pituitary gland and it regulates the ovarian cycle. Not only does this work particularly well for hormone balance but it is a fertility marker.

If you use IF to improve fertility, of course, and you become pregnant, please work with your doctor to change your eating routine to keep your body safe and stable during pregnancy. While IF is not ideal for pregnancy IF has variations and companion eating acceptable styles. For example, healthy fats and limiting refined and processed grains during pregnancy is not only safe-it is strongly suggested!

Many nutritionists prescribe a low carbohydrate and a high-fat diet to those pregnant women who experience gestational diabetes. This example brings home just how healthy and therapeutic these "fasting" model companions are.

Health tips on intermittent fasting for losing weight.

There are many types and methods of intermittent fasting. Just choose one first and try it for a significant period. Skipping on to other methods, again and again, will not help you. Give yourself some time and figure out which method can work best for you. If you have any ongoing medical condition then you should first contact your doctor to avoid the side effects of intermittent fasting. It is important to keep in mind that what you eat is very important and follows small things like sleep well. Add more fiber to your diet, avoid high caloric foods, avoid junk food, and drink enough water. Binging on unhealthy foods overeating days can hamper progress in health.

You should be very clear in your mind first that why are you doing intermittent fasting. If you are doing it just for weight loss then you will have to be more careful about what you eat because you might end up consuming a lot. You must be fasting for a certain period but that doesn't mean that you can go for anything. You should count your maintenance calories and eat less than that to lose weight. If you don't understand this then you should contact a nutritionist who can guide you better.

Make your meal plan. This will help you a lot because you won't be worried about what to eat and when to eat. You can schedule your meals according to the method of fasting that you are going for. There are many benefits of scheduling your meal and designing your meal plan. You get a motivation to stick to your diet and secondly you will not be worried about the whole process of weight loss because you will have a good track of your time and nutrition.

It is important to keep the track of your macronutrients and micronutrients. Even though intermittent fasting has nothing to do with tracking calories but the fact that what you eat sums up into your total calories and they shouldn't exceed your maintenance calories. It is important to eat those foods which have a high nutritional value and try to balance your nutrients. It is better to avoid junk food and concentrate on nutritious food.

The 5: 2 methods. The method spread over the week. It breaks down into five days of healthy eating and two days of fasting. On fasting days, you only entitled to a mini-meal of 500 kcal (a large salad).

The Fasti: It consists of one day of fasting per week, preferably Thursday. You fast 24 hours or more.

You need to do one thing for the initial week. You need to quit breakfast. Why? Two straightforward reasons. Proceed with the fasting around evening time and by skipping breakfast you will generally use less sugar for the day. During this subsequent week, you will proceed not to have breakfast and, additionally, apply two steps that are stopping the additional sugars and Indeed, even the sugars, candy, and aspartame and exclude poor-nutrient starches from lunch.! These are tips that will help you experience the transition better. fasting is challenging at times.

Intermittent Fasting step by step

Intermittent fasting is the act of not eating for a period of 12 to 24 hours.

There are different ways to apply intermittent fasting:

The lean gains method (16h / 8h): It consists of fasting for 16h and being able to eat for 8h. For this, it is enough not to eat breakfast. For example, you finish dinner at 8 p.m., you fast overnight at least noon, nothing prevents you from fasting more if you wish.

The warrior diet: The idea is to eat nothing or little in the morning and noon, then have a big meal in the evening. Physical activity during the "fasting" period is recommended.

The OMAD method (one meal a day) one meal per day: The objective of this method is to prolong the fasting period in one day as much as possible.

Especially at the start. Hunger tends to decrease over time, but some side effects may appear. You might feel many problems like constipation, hypoglycemia, cramps, nutritional deficiencies, etc but you can look for their solutions. It will take time to adapt to this habit but once you will adapt to it you will notice a positive change in your body.

The Best Food And Drinks For Intermittent Fast

Fasting in this segment, let's talk about some foods and the advantages they added in the body in their classes.

HARISSA: This good pasta or chili still has an excellent and perfect reason. The chile is even more widespread in the world, as is believed to have success and protection against cancer.

GET CHEESE: Also, you may feel forgiving, but you got the best of most other cheeses. It also contains the resin, the calcium, and 3% of their daily dose of iron and one-ounce oz.

POPCORN: Popcorn is a high fiber option that your snack list should include.

COCONUT: Coconut is an excellent option to create some wealth. It contains potassium, which can help reduce the risk.

ERED-FED MEAT: Much better is lower at all than what can happen in many other types of meat and higher in some fats, as well as omega-3, monounsaturated fat, etc. It's a great source of iron and protein, which is important for growth and development.

GHEE: Ghee is perfect calcium that is obtained by mixing butter and skimming part of the fat. It also has a slightly pleasant taste. It is rich in vitamins and can use as usual for cooking oils or football.

CANNED SALMON: It is just one of the best foods with vitamin D that is made for health and absorption of calcium.

SPIRULINA: Spirulina is a blue-green alga that is less rich in vitamins, nutrients, and antioxidants that make cells grow. It's a good vegetarian source of protein.

Lemon: This fruit can be acidic to create a light orange scent, but it is equally high in vitamin C, which helps to develop blood cells and that healing is important. Not to mention a small lemon, just for each meal, adds a touch of flavor.

TOFU: Tofu is a great example created by someone and is rich in calcium, protein, and iron.

DANDELION GREENS: The best greens like dandelion are rich in vitamin C and vitamin B, calcium, iron, and potassium.

Purple potatoes: Rich in potassium - you need to care for the heart. What you're special potatoes are about purple color, which comes from anthocyanin, a powerful antioxidant that poses numerous health benefits like one risk lower for cardiovascular disease.

Real recipes: Famous for the crazy good taste (rich in nuts, salty, and somehow supposed) and also for the nutritional punch. Nutrition is also a real recipe with nineteen essential amino acids, such as zinc, selenium, vitamin B, protein, and fiber.

OYSTERS: Oysters are a great choice of protein, in addition to 3 acids, iron, calcium, zinc, and vitamin B12. Vitamin B12 is imminent because it keeps the heart necessary and blessed with good health. Indeed, the data on their precedents are as always shorter.

MAGE: It is a very versatile fruit, with colors that stand out from gray with a reddish red to bright yellow. Also, they are full of vitamins and antioxidants, particularly for vitamin A: all the rest provides 45% of your daily intake.

STRAWBERRIES: They are a good source of vitamin C and other compounds involved in metabolism and also of them.

BLACKBERRIES: Blackberries, in particular, are rich in fiber, which can increase from time to time and satisfied after eating, as are vitamins C, K, and others. The compounds that produce their colors can also vibrate and also boost the immune system.

ARTICHOKES: Some things are much more ecstatic, and herbs are a nutritional potency, a folic acid concentrate, many other fibers, vitamin C, vitamin K and abundant amounts of anhydride, such as quercetin and anthocyanins.

SAUERKRAUT: It ferments one-bit fermentation because it contains multiple fibers and fibers that make an excellent addition to the dining table. Something is a good source of iron, manganese, refrigerant, sodium, magnesium, and calcium. No need to mention the fact that it brings a lot of protein to your diet.

SPAGHETTI SQUASH: Spaghetti has one of the best waters of all winter squashes. It is often found in many and can be used to replace the substance in many responses. Also, a good dose of vitamin A, calcium, vitamin C, and fiber was obtained.

APPLES: There are real reflections and a good idea. Apples are rich in a lot of fiber that still may contain cholesterol, transforming them into one way to start. A little enough to eat apples has allowed people to get at least 15% less than their next meal. One more stupid? They are useful for improving digestion.

WILD CAUGHT: The wild cod can be a variety of vitality and sustainability, which is made possible by them. For body fat, fat is in the form of a-3, also called other cardiovascular risks.

RHUBARB: It is rich in vitamins and fats, as always.

BEET GREENS: It is difficult to understand the correct meaning of beets, but not throw the vegetables that emerge from them. The leaves of some of them, such as paradise and Chiomar vaseline are particularly useful and thought out and can even take into account. They are rich in vitamin A and vitamin K, and one cup contains 44 mg of calcium.

PURPLE CAULIFLOWER: As in many cases, the unexpected shade of this cauliflower comes from the old antioxidant. The cauliflower is in many cases and is fiber, vitamin C, folic acid, vitamin K, and B6 (which always is present in the metabolism and good health). Consider steaming or frying before maintaining high levels of nutrients.

ENDIVE: Endive is rich in inulin and fiber; it can reduce LDL cholesterol levels to improve the situation. Endive is an excellent source of vitamin A and even began as vitamin B, iron, and potassium. Crude often used in some cases, or somehow, it believed that the taste could be pleasant and pleasant.

SNAP PEASE: Small vegetables are ideal snacks because they are rich in nutrients and fiber and have begun to become raw. A good idea as it might seem more - they are dry, they have a pleasant taste. They are also rich in vitamins A, K, and C.

CORN: An ear of corn has the same value as an apple, with all the levels of nutrients nearly always high. It is not still modified; it is often also loaded with lutein and zeaxanthin, two substances that promote health.

PUMPKIN: It appears to be rich in potassium and magnesium, and pumpkin meat is rich in beta-carotene, which is suitable for the immune system. One of these ingredients contains 7 g of fiber and 3 grams of protein, which is useful for regular digestion.

These are some of the foods and drinks which you can add to your meal plan. To know more about such food, check the section below.

Healthy Exercise to support Intermittent Fasting

It is important to have an understanding that what your body wants before going for exercise during intermittent fasting. When you start feeling tired or dizzy, you can experience low blood sugar or become dehydrated. If you experience this then have a drink for a while which is rich in nutrients and then you can have a proper meal later on. Work out and fasting might not go together for some people but many people don't find it comfortable. Before you initiate any diet or exercise program, consult with your doctor or healthcare provider.

If you can do exercise on an empty stomach then you should work out before the window period starts. If you don't like exercising on an empty stomach then between the window period is the most suitable for you. The best choice for success and recuperation is during. Those who like exercising after gaining energy can do it after the window time. Don't forget to keep a track of your macronutrients that you consume before exercise or after having your meal. Time your exercises during your eating cycles is the perfect option for mixing IF and exercise so that your nutritional levels are optimum. And if you're doing the heavy lifting, getting protein after the workout is vital for your body to help with recovery afterward.

Some of the exercises that you can do are given below:

JUMP ROPE: It is a perfect Audio movement; it is also an excellent correct movement. It also helps and strengthens muscles, increases fitness, and burns many calories in a small period.

QUICK FEET

Also, if your goodwill is the improvement in your mood and good sense, and get a good cardio pulse during the cycle, try to make sure that your feet remain train.

ALPINESTARS

Mountain sports are the right compound exercise and a powerful reinforcement everywhere.

BREEDING OF THE SEAT SCHOLARSHIP

It helps in strengthening the inner side, thighs, and calves. One more reason is tears, and even thoughts maintain balance.

REVERSED BOARD

Envying the case is one exercise of enormous scope that strengthens its core, glutes, weight, thighs, and others. If you have decided to put everything in your body for work, it improves stability and flexibility and enhances metabolism.

BASKETBALL SHOT

The fact is that it is a high level, because the whole body improves and adapts, develops strength, and also increases speed and coordination.

TOUCH AND HOPE

The best way is a cardio-filled movement that challenges your strength and stability and improves durability, courage, and skill. It allowed us to narrow the legs, increase the dose, and lose weight.

Ankle jump

The ankle maintains the tone and carves things, squeezes the heart, and also triggers the aerobic form. This opportunity also increases your skill, coordination, and attention.

CALF HEIGHTS

This exercise allows you to increase muscle strength, everything you want to enhance and improve the appearance, definition, and appearance of the latter.

SQUAT BECERRO AGING

The right place for calf rearing is a great exercise to give you the strength of your buttocks and legs. This exercise aimed at the people most affected by others, their calves, but try to maintain a squat.

Healthy Recipes For Intermittent Fasting

These recipes are low-calorie recipes that you can enjoy with your fast, which will leave you full of feeling.

LIGHTER CREAMY MUSHROOMS IN TOAST

Surely and luxuriously, you will never think that this breakfast is only 200 kcal and counts as one of your five.

BANANA MUFFIN:

Ripped added to muffins accordingly, so you don't have to use juice. While flour gives muffins a lot of fiber, it keeps you full at all times.

OMELETTE OF GARLIC MUSHROOMS:

The pleasure and music will bring great excitement to last this to reduce calories, even to make a tortilla.

CHICKEN BALLS AND VEGETABLES:

Try this grilled chicken and balti to get a delicious recipe that is quick and easy to prepare.

Crispy Banana and Yogurt:

Cream and yogurt are a perfect combination of low calories that will help you spend the night. Goodness had to say it without the need for a first extract, and the seeds bring a satisfying crunch. As part of an intermittent diet.

CAPONATA RATATOUILLE:

It is rarely a wrapping vegetable that has been able to give rise to the origin of Provence. Perfect for satisfying pleasantly and making people eat too.

ITALIAN STYLE MEATBALLS WITH TAGLIATELLE DE ZUCCHINI:

This flat flavorful of Italian meatballs have a healthy twist by using coquette ribbons instead of pasta an easy way to reduce calories.

CHERMOULA TOFU AND ROASTED VEGETABLES:

By luck, he has also been able to express the flavors of this taste. Serve with freshly cut vegetables for a hearty vegetarian meal.

YOGUR-BERRY:

Apparently, as a fruitful fruit that is an excellent satisfactory choice, the use of frozen berries makes it a right suspect, they think.

VEGETABLE SOUP FOR THE HEART:

This abundant, velvety soup is full of goodness and goodness, perfect to meet on a cold night. If you eat on a short day with an intermittent diet, replace the pieces with unnecessary ones for each day.

LAMB AND FLAGELLET LAMB BEANS:
It was a perfect way to fill your cold. Do not waste time, and this is enough for you to help you comply.

CHERRY PACK AND CHERRY FISH:
Make the fish as it is a great way to recover energy. Give the first and the other meat with the chili and cilantro.

Pork sautéed with ginger and soy sauce:
This little and uncomfortable little pig is fast, and it may be that everything continues to lose flavor and help you have fun.

To get the full recipes to check out the section below.

Intermittent Fast And Keto: Should You Combine The Two?

The intermittent fasting and keto diet are two of the most popular wellness developments of the day. The ketogenic diet method (keto) will likely be a superior approach to body fat and decreasing carbohydrate content. Intermittent fasting can help the human body become ketosis much faster than the keto diet program alone. It is the main reason why the body, during fasting, maintains its energy balance by shifting its source of energy from carbohydrates to fats - the basic principle of the prepared keto diet.

Combining the ketogenic diet with intermittent fasting is probably safe for many people. On the other hand, pregnant women and those who have a history of disorderly care should avoid intermittent fasting.

It seems that this is happening and what to do to cut and think you want, there are countless ideas. You may have some ideas on how to perform, get on your cardio, and eat well. Perhaps you have already had three of these. However, many people do not have/ never had anything like flashing. Right?

Fasting is an ancient ritual, which has been followed over the centuries by many cultures and religions. To treat obesity intermittent fasting was used as a therapeutic tool in 1915. Intermittent fasting was observed for 1-14 days in the initial period. This excitement entered lay magazines which encouraged researchers and clinicians to be careful about using intermittent fasts without medical supervision. The 5:2 diet, a new kind of intermittent fasting started in the UK in 2012.

You can try so many strategies to minimize your calories and remain in a calorie deficit to improve your health and reduce your weight. It seems like something is happening and there are endless suggestions about what to do to cut and what you like. You may have some thoughts on exercising, getting on your cardio, and eating well. You might have tried all three strategies but still, they are not helpful to some people. The question is how the concept of intermittent fasting was derived?

Even before the advent of great ancient cultures, the benefits of intermittent fasting were reaped by hunter-gatherers all over the world. There are written records that are evidence that humans used 'starvation' to help their body heal and enjoy the health benefits it provided. Various ancient cultures, independent of territory or religion, used intermittent fasting and were well aware of its efficacy.

Periodic fasting was used not just to cure the illnesses in ancient Egypt, Greece but also to prevent many diseases. Intermittent fasting was highly common in the Middle Ages as people sought to enjoy its benefits.

But our ancestors, hunter-gatherers, practiced intermittent fasting long before the ancient Egyptians, Greek, and Hindu, because of food shortages. Before agriculture, when they came home empty-handed, people consumed what they could find, and wild berries were found nowhere, periods of famine took place, and this helped strengthen hunter-gatherers. This activity also played a key role in almost all the major religions of the world, as it was synonymous with penance and other forms of self-control.

When we take a closer look at the past of various religions and their relation with intermittent fasting. The Judaism and has several common behaviors that include Yom Kippur, the truth of some; In Islam, he died very quickly during April, while once again and even later, he lost 40 times during Lent, the period in which Christ fasted to 40 in the desert. Muslims also practice fasting during the month of Ramadan.

They must have had about ten for the preparation religious, known as good anorexia (lack of appetite miraculous); Surviving for carefree adults has been recognized as a hallmark of holiness and security.

Giuliana Norwich, an English anchor and a myth that lived in the fifteenth part used as a means of communication with Christ.

In other systems belief, the gods thought to offer the divine reveal their teaching in dreams and visions only after a fast of temple priests. Also another for a reason, one can see from the aspect politics, the fasting gesture long has also been used as one political protest. The classic example Mahatma Gandhi undertook is suffragettes 17 fasts during the struggle for the independence of India: his longest lasted 21 days. But the election has also had the positive side, having been exploited by exhibitionists and adventurers, and they took into account.

Intermittent fasting is the most common debate these days and so scientists are busy collecting data regarding intermittent fasting. Harvard conducted research recently which showed that Intermittent fasting increases the life expectancy of an individual practicing it as it improves health.

Harvard experts have found that by altering mitochondrial networks inside cells — either through dietary restriction or by mimicking genetic manipulation — an individual may expand their survival and help to improve health.

Fasting is an old and time-tested tradition. It was not only used for weight loss but also to boost focus, prolong life, prevent Alzheimer's disease, prevent insulin resistance, and even undo the whole aging process. Rather than trying some new, never-before-tried diet cure, we should concentrate on past ancient healing rituals. Practically every culture and religion on earth followed this approach.

There's always the same eye-rolling reaction when speaking of fasting. A Hunger? Is that the answer? No. No. Fasting is a whole different type of beast. Starvation is the unintended shortage of food. It is not intentional, nor regulated.

Those individuals who are starving are never sure about their meal like when will they get their next meal. On the other hand, fasts are voluntarily refusing food for moral, nutritional, or other purposes. Both terms have a different meaning and they shouldn't be confused. Fasting can be performed for any period, from a couple of hours to months on end. Fasting is one way or another is a component of daily life. The word 'break easily' is the meal breaking the fast – which is done every day.

Fasting is a very old practice followed by many people.. Hippocrates Cos is generally regarded as the founder of modern medicine. Among the therapies, he recommended and advocated was fasting exercise and apple cider vinegar intake. Plutarch the very famous writer and historian of the ancient Greek times also believed that fasting is better than taking medication.

The ancient Greeks thought fasting would improve cognitive abilities. You must have noticed this that after eating a heavy meal or after consuming more than your maintenance calories like on occasions you don't feel healthy or energetic and instead you feel tired and lazy. The latter is more probable. To deal with the enormous influx of food, blood is funneled into the digestive system, and so less blood is left for the brain. Food coma results.

I'm deviating a bit to show the obesity problems that can be created by preparing. And how to get there for these problems. In the past, obesity has ceased or ceased to exist and do the same. It has more widespread responses, which spread even further in the same way. Although the prevention of massive budgets and the reason is political, policy and truth have also been far dangerously multiplying.

It's beginning in society has not yet found a point that experts have started to call it "discreetly," one of what was said for the first time, regardless of its development.

Recent studies have shown that a high level of success has had some excess associated with excess weight, reaching more than 300 million worldwide. The weapon was explained just before when childhood & youth obesity was assumed. These nutritional disorders involve some of these associated with other cases, some of them chronic, even if they are of a different type, as already mentioned, high blood levels and others even more prevalent. Obesity repeated it, as previously mentioned since people have had the most continued to develop in this way—all in proper doses of good and a considerable recovery throughout life.

They strive to produce outcomes while speaking about all therapies, which can sometimes incorporate therapeutic techniques and tools before they start. Bearing in mind some World Health Organization (WHO) figures, the cause of death of 41 million of the 64 million people who died in 2015 collapsed. Although it is associated with some cause, in this case even with hypertension, but also with the most severe syndrome, it is likely to result in 80%.

It is important to make a strategy to cope up with the increasing percentage of obesity worldwide. obesity and hypertension are major risk factors of so many diseases. It is important to fight this problem. Multiple disciplinary professionals are required to help the organization by providing solutions about the current health problem.

The team of professionals includes primary health care doctors, progressive Extermination, nutritionists, psychologists, and specialized doctors. Strengthening their invasion and creating a healthy life by trying to restore this situation is the responsibility of all the social actors involved. Returning to flogging, most of the truth had a religious purpose.

Fasting is the perfect way to improve your insulin sensitivity. Insulin levels are lowered by intermittent fasting and this way the need for insulin is altered positively. The insulin levels are raised all the time on becoming immune to insulin and the body will keep on wanting to transfer the sugar into your fat cells and this will result in drowsiness, cold temperature, and exhaustion. That is the real issue. Two things depend on resistance. It's not just the high levels but those levels' durability.

What people have learned is that insulin resistance, because it relies on those two factors, can weaken the resistance and it breaks your stability, a period where you can get the insulin levels very down. Not only the levels but those levels' durability. The fastest, cleverest, most reliable way to fast is intermittent fasting. If you follow a short type of intermittent fasting then it means that you will be consuming all the food at one time which should be consumed at different times of the day. In short, intermittent fasting means you are eating all the food you are going to consume in a limited amount of time in a day. People are fast everywhere, depending on the targets, from 12-20 hours a day. Even intermittent fasting is one of the best ways to restore your sensitivity to insulin.

Apart from controlling blood sugar, eating just one meal one day brings more several benefits – reducing size waist, increasing muscle through increased HGH hormone assuming that the individual does not meal void of proteins, reduced blood pressure, improved lipid profile through lower LDL / Shoot, and higher HDL, reduced CRP or inflation, sound, even earlier, more significant with time as in any case, and so on. In some religions, time is a way to purify and corroborate the body and is considered safe. The fasting can also use to reduce or lose sight according to what was said.

People use drinking like a guy to detoxify their bodies to him. For some time, certain examinations or certain surgical procedures may be required until the course lasts throughout the fasting period. Therefore, the idea of fasting that also makes it more compelling in this situation, the best way will not be with any diet that would appear. In any event, catering isn't necessarily what happens, but that's what most people say when they listen to it.

Having the food, however, is not a sin, above. For some decades, as in many others, the small concept of correcting is to recover from a right option in some years. But in this sense, you might choose to describe fasting as behaving – in return for dietary habits rather than three square meals a day or a handful of smaller day meals during when you're in a particular period, in either case, it's a few days of the day.

You should know what you did during that time, too. Of course, by definition, you would consume it. If you eat the same, it is unlikely that you will be looking for the qualities of the preparation.

But if you practice fasting and stick a diet mostly whole, rich in fruits, vegetables, lean proteins, healthy fats, and raw food dairy, you are changed and for those occasional splurges in chocolate or cheese would not have as much of one impact as you would if you were one diet calorie-restrictive- That the beauty of fasting is right there in one way to do it. Several types are there. Let's take a look at your brand.

Different types of intermittent fasting

1. The intimate fasting: This is why it is also called cyclic fasting.

   Intermittent administration is an excellent phrase to eat (and not do) intact. After all accounts, almost all the best methods among those that follow are those of intimate fasting! Typical fast intermediate times between 14 and 18 hours. The rest of the period in which one or other of these things would come out of your case could be 32 to 36 days.

2. Using time-limited: If you are taking a timely break, start doing between 12 and 16 hours for all. You can consume as many of your favorite nutritious foods as you want during this period. It is one of the most important. The timely response is merely inevitable in light of what has been produced. First, if dinner finishes at 7 p.m., you can't do something until 7 p.m. You can extend the remaining time until around 11.00 or 12.00 if you desire to proceed further. If you don't get enough sleep. After eating, it is a way to introduce your passion to your lifestyle and experiences with everyone. It is a different name for the limited start time, here you

will have to continue for 16-hour each day and then eat the other eight.

3. Before beginning each day, alternating the day you managed to minimize the number of calories you consume for the next few days and then consume enough for each day. The path is also not feasible but will aim to get around 25 for around its average calorie intake. For eg, some people to eat in 2000 would have been reduced by about 500 to 500. Furthermore, fasting is not inherently a long-term strategy as it can be difficult to prove, but it can be useful to get a good habit on the move.

4. The fast Dannio: This is very similar to what he has always done well because he never gets enough five times a week. On the other hand, two are limited to around 500-600 calories per day—a further example of preparation. If so, it will stick to fruits and vegetables during the day and then eat a little bigger, more prominent in the

world. It is a small spiritual fast. Starting from Damian, he well accommodated in Denise's Bible's Beckon; Dannie Fast is a real start concerning vegetables, fruits, and others, still healthy and healthy, but they are anyway. And the drinks you want, too, and the juice avoided. Most people know the following for another 21 days before starting a good experience, also to make it even stronger. The claim has been a good idea of what has been created for thousands of years. Although we should continue with it and much more mind-body, fasting is doing a great success because of all their benefits. There may be one impending slowdown of the reaction, and the 3 (three) supported scientifically ready to restore the immune system. Breastfeeding may have some benefits, and also the fasting can be beneficial for weight, but like all things, and in any case, there is still something to do. The women probably want to do more to consider the idea of using time as a useful tool.

Intermittent fasting consists of reducing calories as much as possible during a given period so that the body, deprived of energy, will then draw on its reserves, first of sugars, then of fats, to lose weight. Fasting can be practiced in different ways.

There are several types of intermittent fasting, which vary according to the actual fasting time, and according to the feeding window to follow:

Daily fasting (16/8 method):
It is a question of fasting during 16h, then to concentrate all your meals on a period of 8h, to then fast again. It is the strategy most used, in particular by Hugh Jackman, to prepare his role for Wolverine.

The times you choose don't matter as long as you stick to the two periods of fasting and eating. However, it is much easier to fast when you sleep (hours pass faster).

The weekly fast (eat-stop-eat):
If you are afraid to start a daily fast, you can start with the weekly fast, which consists of not eating for 24 hours, once a week. For example, you can eat breakfast one morning and then not eat until the next morning.

Intermittent fasting every other day:
Fasting either two days a week (during which only about a quarter of the usual calories are consumed), a method called the 5: 2 diet;
On other days, we usually eat, "to the full," without any obligation to monitor ourselves particularly (but also without "gorging").

It is merely a question of fasting 24 hours every other day. This style of fasting is generally the least practiced by aficionados of intermittent fasting but is nevertheless the alternative of "intermittent fasting," which is most often used in scientific studies.

When you fast alternately, you eat NOTHING?
For the first two methods (1 day on 2 or 2 days per week), you can either eat nothing except a few broths (strict approach) or eat extremely light, around only 25% of the daily calories needed (450 kcal maximum, to consume ideally around 12-14h).

For the "fasting," it is enough, in reality, to dine early (before 8 p.m.), and to skip breakfast to start eating only at noon minimum: we are finally satisfied with spacing the meals (we can ultimately make three meals over these 8 hours, for example, 12 p.m., 4 p.m., and 7:30 p.m., even if, usually, we are content with two).

This strategy would allow the body to detoxify, burn fat, but also to benefit from other benefits that we will list below.

Why these variations, and which one to choose? Challenging question. The first method was popularized by Martin Berkhan, who makes it the primary tool of his fitness method, which would allow gaining muscle mass while losing fat weight.

The other versions of intermittent fasting based on 24-hour fasting, and illustrate the theory that the longer the fast, the more beneficial effects are observed.

If you want to test "intermittent fasting," be sure to choose the strategy that seems most suitable for you and the one that you will manage to respect and carried out the test over one month.

First of all: what is fasting?

You know for sure that you are happy holding the meal to the right end.

Considered the truth, this is only difficult for three days, but the mileage varies. The intimate fasting (IF) is a bit different and involves a short period of 12-16 days. Most of us are healthy every night between dinner and breakfast every day, but in the meantime, fitted (IF) is a bit easier. Some only managed for 8 (eight) windows during the day; someone has to do at least 24 and others only for a cold, windy night. It opens a step when does the intermittent fasting.

Intermittent fasting has like benefits, and these will be culminating and, therefore, will reach more than 12 hours, as it has promising health benefits. It might help to prolong the life of every advantage. You can also determine glucose levels, a good selection of fluids, a little mass, and help you lose weight. You can improve the entire turnover, reduce inflammation, and aid in proper rehabilitation.

It can also slow down the aging process: during the recruitment phase, the cells die, and some are activated, although this is still time again and repeated.

A brilliant idea for some people is that a lot 'of 12 + of the time without food for their body; happily, at night, it's easier to detoxify and rehabilitate. Often, holding stored for fuel is necessary when you're fasting on your own. The aim to do so, however, is not the best for us.
Everyone else may consider that it is entirely different from religion, and any other mention at the beginning.

What are the after-effects of intermittent fasting?

The heart of the matter. Why deprive us of food on such vast time slots? The main answer is simple and fits the goal that many people want to achieve: weight loss.

Researchers are studying fasting mainly because it is an alternative to the ranking factors for fighting obesity, which is physical activity and modification of diet, and the diseases linked to it.

Indeed, it is not a question of playing sports or of ceasing to eat such or such food, but to concentrate the meals on strict time slots, and to respect periods of fasting. Great, right?

Since the early 2000s, numerous studies have carried out, and the results of intermittent fasting have been generally positive. Among other things, this strategy would:

Why use fasting to lose weight?

The short answer is that it works; on top of that, fasting has many health benefits.

Obesity has always existed, and it can say that it is increasing as fast as the number of pounds of diet.

The subject is therefore not new, and there are thousands of methods, more or less active, for losing weight.

So why choose intermittent fasting? When they sell their dung, certain media qualify to fast as a simple, fashionable diet that will run its course as others do, then will disappear. Here's why fasting is becoming more and more popular. Over the past 30-year, numerous scientific studies have demonstrated its benefits and superiority over low-calorie diets.

It's better than a diet

At the point when you need to shed pounds, you should realize that it is hypothetically challenging to get in shape without losing muscle. All the better you can do is limit muscle decrease to enhance fat loss. Sports, nourishment, and fasting can get you there. This research equates the loss of weight from fasting with low-calorie intakes. Fasting permits you to lose weight as well, but it protects your muscles better, which implies that you lose an increased amount of fat.

Fasting improves the creation of the growth hormone required for the growth of muscles, so it is a generally excellent approach to accelerate muscle gain.

It diminishes hunger

Another point that truly recognizes fasting from slims down diet plans is its effect on appetite and longings. During the initial week, an increased sensation of hunger felt. However, by the second week, it starts reducing and continues with the increase of time.

It has been commonly demonstrating that diets increment the feeling of yearning; it is connected to the effect on two hormones that control appetite and satiety: leptin and ghrelin. I will disclose to you how fasting is having a much-improved impact on these hormones and subsequently will cause you to get more fit while diminishing your craving.

The impact on leptin

Our fat produces a hormone called Leptin; it regulates our metabolism and tells our brain that we must stop eating; it is the hormone of satiety. Leptin decreases drastically after a low-calorie diet. The amount of leptin in the blood is regulated over the long term by the amount of fat in our body, the more we have, the more leptin we have. Therefore, if we lose our fat, we have less leptin, it causes increased hunger.

It also applies to fat loss with fasting. Fasting, however, counteracts this effect with spikes in leptin triggered by the breaking of the fast. Leptin is also regulated over the short term by the quantities of food that we eat.

The intermittent fasting makes it possible to have high peaks of leptin during the breaking of the fast. It allows you to counterbalance its decline in the rest of the day. It is not the case with a low-calorie diet, and our body is permanent with lower leptin, which increases the feeling of hunger.

The impact on ghrelin
Ghrelin is the other hormone that regulates hunger and is secreted by the brain, stomach, and intestine. This scientific study shows that it generally emits before the meals we usually eat. It is as if it is preparing our body to digest or reminds us that it is soon time to eat. However, with fasting, ghrelin gradually decreases. So be less and less hungry before your usual meals. Ghrelin levels vary depending on the level of insulin in the body. The drop in insulin level during the young could explain the decline in ghrelin.

Hunger linked to habit

Some people who practiced this reported that beyond the impact of ghrelin, concretely, it was noticed that desire manifests itself at the same time as when they ate "normally." At 11 a.m., noon, around 4 p.m., and 7 p.m. After two weeks of fasting, only hunger for noon and 7 p.m. appeared. Also, by drinking a glass of lukewarm water or herbal tea, the feeling of hunger disappears.

Fasting will allow you to decondition yourself in some way. It is true liberation. Today after several months of intermittent fasting, I feel real freedom from hunger and food.

Improved insulin sensitivity

The first factor that will determine whether you store fat or not is the level of insulin in your blood. Contrary to what all diet gurus say, the number of calories is only secondary.

For example, people with type 1 diabetes may eat 5,000k calories a day, and they will not store fat because they have little or no insulin in the blood.

Fasting is the most effective and longest-lasting method to tackle this chronic rise in insulin and restore insulin sensitivity.

It's practical and economical
When we fast we eat less often, so we free up a lot of time that we usually spent cooking and eating.

The other practical aspect is its simplicity. The rules are simple. Just eat nothing or drink caloric drinks for more than 12 hours.

Specialist Jason Fung has attempted a great deal to assist his diabetic patients with changes in their dietary patterns. Notwithstanding, not many patients prepared to change their lifestyle, particularly elderly patients. With fasting, he finds a greatly improved appropriation and foundation of propensity by patients. It is more straightforward because it doesn't request that they alter the nourishment they eat, yet just the times of eating.

It appears to be a lot simpler to embrace and follow over the long haul. Dr. Fung has helped several patients recuperate from type 2 diabetes.

However, if you have a diabetic patient and need to do fasting, you should approach your physician for counseling, he will most likely alter your treatment downwards to evade hypoglycemia since fasting brings typically down your glucose level.

Autophagy

In 2016 the Nobel Prize in Medicine was awarded to a Japanese researcher who demonstrated the value of autophagy, a mechanism possible only during fasting. Autophagy allows our bodies to recycle unnecessary and damaged things in our cells. The young person, therefore, will enable you to activate a real body makeover.

High blood pressure

Fasting is one of the most effective and super simple ways to lower blood pressure. Several scientific studies validate this point.

Intermittent fasting and hormones

Women are more responsive to intermittent fasting than men because they have more kisspeptin, which is linked to reproductive functions and creates greater sensitivity to fasting.

The hormones which regulate reproductive functions are highly sensitive to the hormones of hunger. An experiment conducted on female rats found that disrupting their reproductive hormones took only 15 days of eating every second day. The experiment continued for 2 weeks, which is a 10 year equivalent for humans. Fasting may have a similar effect on women. A female's hormones are very closely intertwined with their metabolism.

Fasting's effect on women isn't just about having more kisspeptin. Furthermore, women are more sensitive to cortisol, which increases during fasting. Cortisol is a stress hormone with desirable fat-burning properties, but it can also cause female hormonal imbalances. Its adrenal gland releases cortisol. It helps to control the levels of blood sugar, regulate your metabolism, and reduce inflammation.

Intermittent fasting and other fasting methods are known to help correct the hormones of hunger and blood sugar. Fasting enhances insulin sensitivity and enhances metabolism. Fasting won't make you feel hungry in the long run, as opposed to continuous calorie restriction. Instead, it increases the levels of leptin and adiponectin, thus improving the sensation of satiety. Also, it affects the hunger hormone ghrelin and enhances the levels of dopamine (the happy hormone).

Fasting and intermittent fasting can cause a drop in the levels of your T3 thyroid hormone, which will resume to its normal level once you start eating again. You need to consider your entire HPA (Hypothalamic Pituitary Adrenal) axis when considering the impact of the fasting on your thyroid health. It's your brain, your thyroid, and your adrenal glands communicating. The hormonal changes that occur at fasting all work in harmony together as a whole.

A drop in the T3 hormone may not be such a bad thing to compensate for the lack of glucose and the production of ketones. When you fast, your body heals itself as it starts producing ketones in the process of autophagy. Well, that's how you get your hormones corrected.

What about the elderly woman? When practicing intermittent fasting, are there certain factors to consider? Well, for one thing, intermittent fasting slows the process of aging, which I'm sure most older women will be happy to hear. Also, aging women tend to struggle with weight gain, and intermittent fasting will help keep a healthy weight going. Insulin resistance is an important factor contributing to hot flashes. Intermittent fasting will help to reduce the hot flashes and many other uncomfortable symptoms for the menopausal woman. Maintaining your insulin level stable after menopause is equally essential.

It may help prevent weight gain, reduce inflammation, and improve your hormonal health.

What you don't want to like? Intermittent fasting can be beneficial for women of all ages. However, learning how to practice intermittent fasting safely is important. Intermittent fasting is not just about leaving breakfast. There are many approaches, some involve an overnight fast for just 12 hours. Some, like fasting at the crescendo, require fasting every second day for 14-16 hours. Other intermittent fasting approaches are about fasting for a whole day or lowering your calorie intake twice a week to 500 per day.

Intermittent fasting most suitable for women, why?

Females are seen as more sensitive to calorie restriction and so the effects of intermittent fasting will be different in men and women. The sensitivity can also affect hormone levels and can also cause changes in the menstrual cycle. Because of fasting for a longer period or very often the function of the hypothalamus can be impaired as hormones that regulate the menstrual cycle are regulated by the hypothalamus. This is the reason why women need a modified sort of approach. They can consider alternated days of fasting, or fasting for shorter periods.

Hormones go out of balance when women restrict their calories, their metabolism slows down, and the body cannot function at their optimal levels.

So if you're a woman who limits her calories and intermittent fasting, you're doing more harm than good to your body and you're missing the benefits of intermittent fasting.

Incorporated in a weight loss program, intermittent fasting can be beneficial for women as the body continues to receive the nutrients it needs. Knowing that intermittent fasting can have different effects on women of different ages, is important.

Who should not invade to start?

The best way to start fasting is a few days a week. It means that you do not need to invade yourself in intermittent fasting every two days, only two or three days at a time. You should be able to do it for 12-16 hours (point to 14-16), which is not that difficult. It occurs to you to eat after dinner at 7 μm and, therefore, do not repeat everything until seven at night. First, if it is difficult for you in the beginning then you can try to do it often, 5-7 days at a time. It also had a great start to a 24-hour flood. There are many different options; you need to see what works for you.

When should you avoid the intense reaction?
The intimate fasting is not the right choice for everyone. You should not consider intermittent fasting if you are: pregnant or nursing under chronic stress; one has previous history disordered of eating such as bulimia or anorexia, struggle with sleep disorders, or have difficulty sleeping.

How does intermittent fasting work?
Intermittent fasting, often called IF, will not force you to starve yourself. It also does not permit you to eat tons of unhealthy food during the period you're not fasting. Instead of eating all-day meals and snacks, you're eating within a specific period.

Some people think It has succeeded for them simply because the small eating window of course allows them to minimize the number of calories they consume. For example, they may find that instead of consuming 3 meals and 2 snacks, they only have time for 2 meals and one snack. They become more aware of the types of food they eat and tend to remain away from processed carbs, unhealthy fat, and empty calories.

You can, of course, choose the kinds of healthy food you love too. While some people opt to lower their overall intake of calories, others combine IF with a keto, vegan, or another diet. These are some metabolic changes caused by IF which could help to account for synergistic benefits. The lower insulin levels will help improve fat burning during the fasting period. While the levels of insulin decrease, the levels of HGH increase to promote fat burning and muscle development.

In response to an empty belly, Noradrenaline will be sent to cells by the nervous system to let them know they need to release fat for the fuel.

What to be careful?
Is periodic fasting Safe? Know that you can only last for 12 to 16 hours, and not for days at a time. You still have plenty of time to enjoy a balanced and fulfilling diet. Some older women can need to eat regularly, due to metabolic disorders or medication instructions. In any situation, you can speak to your health care provider about your eating habits before making any adjustments.

However, not everyone has needs during fasting. But it is true that at least one night of fasting for at least 10 hours to allow your body to repair it alone while studying. It can't happen when it's a night when you have a lot of good things to digest. That is right people who did not explain well when they have had great success and have done.

If you have tired adrenals or hypoglycemia, or you cannot sleep through the night, you may need a small before bed snack to support blood sugar, and that is a sign that you should work on regulating blood sugar and nourishing your hormones before you can successfully.

Although advocates boast the euphoric-like benefits that they experience from restricted eating times, very little if anything discussed in current research about the impacts of intermittent fasting on women's health, particularly hormones, the female brain, energy, and long-term benefits and or consequences.

Fasting is a great way to keep your body and mind and perfectly clean. The minimum adrenaline in your body also increases in the case of a short-term onset, but your body can burn to burn and overload and work harder. Think about this with the increased metabolism, and see how you can lose weight that could be caused by intermittent administration.

Intermittent fasting is considered as a trend for some people:

Many diet and exercise trends originate in legitimate science, although the facts tend to distort when they reach first popularity. The benefits were exaggerated, and the risks were minimized. Science ranks second in the market. So popular that it is rushing in the territory of fashion, suggests Pilon. And when something becomes a prevalent trend, but only for a short time, there are usually several problems.

On the one hand, he says, many doctors and nutrition experts are inclined to rule out fashion. Then, their patients and clients, while being protected from the ridiculous claims of evangelists too jealous in the diet, can also lose the legitimate benefits of a well-done fast. Another concern is that promoters of the intermittent fasting, perhaps without realizing it, will encourage extreme behavior, such as binge eating. The implication is that if you fast two days a week, you can eat all the garbage in your esophagus, you can swallow for the remaining five days. Not so, say more moderate supporters of fasting.

Your opinion on intermittent fasting:
And in most cases, in a reasonable way, do not eat anything for a prolonged period from time to time, and consent only occasionally (maybe once a week, for example, on a specific day).

There is research, they argue, to support the health benefits of the sensible incorporation of fasting into your lifestyle. There is a great deal of research that helps the health benefits of fasting, although most have done in animals, not humans. However, the results have been promising. The fasting has shown to improve biomarkers of disease, reduce oxidative stress and preserve learning and memory performance, according to Mark Mattson, chief researcher at the National Institute on Aging, part of the National Institutes of health.

Mattson studied the health benefits of intermittent fasting in the cardiovascular system and the brain in rodents and requested "well-controlled human studies in people" through a series of body mass indices. There are several theories which provide fast physiological benefits, says Mattson. "What we have studied a lot and designed experiments to test is the hypothesis that cells are under mild stress during the fasting period," he says. The NDE respond adaptively to stress by improving their ability to cope with stress and, perhaps, to resist disease.

Although the word stress is often used in a negative sense, taxing the body and mind has benefits. Consider intense exercise, which emphasizes the muscles and the cardiovascular system in particular. The extent of your body time to recover, get stronger.

"There is a striking similarity between how cells respond to exercise stress and how cells respond to intermittent fasting," says Mattson. Mattson has contributed to numerous other studies on intermittent fasting and caloric restriction. In one, overweight adults with moderate asthma have consumed only 20% of their regular calorie intake every two days. Participants who have adhered to the diet lost 8% of their initial body weight for eight weeks. They also saw a decrease in oxidative stress and inflammation markers and an improvement in asthma-related symptoms and several indicators of quality of life.

In another study, Mattson and colleagues explored the effects of intermittency and energy restriction continues in weight loss and various biomarkers (for conditions such as breast cancer, diabetes, and cardiovascular disease) between WOM overweight young and n. They found that intermittent restriction was as useful as one restriction continuous improvement weight loss, insulin sensitivity, and other biomarkers for health.

Mattson also studied the protective benefits of fasting for neurons. If you do not eat for 10-16 hours, in which your body enters its fat stores for fatty acids and energy called ketones released into the bloodstream. It has shown to protect memory and learning functionality, says Mattson, as well as slowing pathological processes in the brain. But perhaps it is not so much fasting that produces health benefits, per se, as the consequent general reduction in calorie intake (in this case, you do not overeat on days without fasting, which could generate an excess of calories instead of a deficit).

The caloric restriction without malnutrition is the only experimental approach consistently demonstrated for prolonged survival in animal models, Freedland and his colleagues have said in a study of the effects of intermittent fasting on the growth of prostate cancer in mice. In the study, mice fasted twice a week for 24 hours, but otherwise, they were allowed to eat freely. On rest days, mice overestimate. In general, they have not lost weight, counteracting the benefits they could have seen from fasting. The study concluded that intermittent fasting with overeating compensatory did not improve mouse survival, nor retarded the growth of the prostate tumor.

If you want to improve your health, the goal should be to lose weight by reducing the total amount of calories consumed, Freedland suggests, rather than focusing on when these calories are consumed. "If you don't eat two days a week and limit what you eat for the other five days, you will lose weight. It is a weight loss approach, he says. "I'm not sure if it works better than reducing a short seven days a week.

Intermittent Fasting in Women and Menopause:

Intermittent fasting for menopausal and postmenopausal women is having great results. In post-menopause research, women lose twice as much weight as premenopausal women because of poorer dietary adherence. These findings suggest that after menopause fasting can be of particular benefit to women.

Intermittent fasting is also an effective way of reducing abdominal fat and avoiding weight gain before and after menopause. It can also help reduce diabetes risk by reducing cholesterol, blood pressure, and insulin resistance. Both types of intermittent fasting work, so you can choose the approach that best fits your lifestyle and stick to it for a long time.

Intermittent fasting benefits for women

1. It helps improve the body's metabolism and the ability to burn fat in the short term. Periodic fasting has shown to reduce fat preserve lean mass muscle in both men and women as it boosts the human growth factor.
2. Just like exercise, stress helps you build a fitter body. Hard times make you stronger, and winter cold helps us appreciate the heat summer; fasting periods can provide you with a chance to have an opportunity to enjoy. Between meals, followed by a good dose of food and replenishment. Take advantage of a really (eating) window, in which you can fully drink and digest the food you have consumed.
3. You may have had common problems during and after showing how effective it has been for blood regulation

and improvement, especially concerning food and fish. (Arnn later, 2017). A review of some individuals who have to fast than those who began studying found that others started improving insulin.

4. Improves Sugar in the Blood: Glucose is the simplified form of complex carbohydrates. When the food is ingested glucose is absorbed by the body. Insulin is released by the pancreas which transfers the glucose from the bloodstream to the cells where it can be utilized. Insulin doesn't work properly in diabetic patients and so they have high blood sugar which also causes symptoms in diabetic patients like increased thirst, hunger, and urination, etc. Intermittent fasting maintains the sugar level and prevents crashes and spikes.

5. The first is the fasting process that causes leptin and ghrelin to be formed which are the hormones of hunger. But, as women

offer some period of intermittent fasting, they report in the long run feeling less hungry. The second element in women's intermittent fasting is that fasting impairs reproductive capability, so fasting is not recommended for pregnant women. Fertility issues will appear if women will not consume sufficient calories or proper nutrition. But if IF is handled properly there is no need to think about it. Some women may also increase their fertility after losing some extra weight.

6. With age, the metabolism slows down. While fewer calories are needed to hold the weight of women over 40 years old. Women over 40 are typically exposed to pre- and post-menopausal periods and the deposition of fat in the midsection is increased. It is difficult to lose belly fat and it is linked with many complications such as high cholesterol levels, raised blood pressure, and type II diabetes.

Intermittent fasting to prevent such problems is an excellent way to keep you fit and safe. Intermittent fasting helps in reducing belly fat and the reason is the production of human growth hormone which aids in fat loss. The levels of HGH increase when the insulin content is low. Low insulin in turn will increase the HGH and this will result in increased burning of fat. To achieve good results try to do exercise, take good sleep, and fast.

Stress and balance factors

We experience many stresses every day and fasting is also like a stressor. It creates an effect similar to that of exercise on the body, yelling at others, running from predators, or being stressed. When the body is not able to handle the intermittent fasting it will create problems. This can have negative results if taken too far.

What to do today

Here are some things which make your body's fasting less stressful:

- Getting adapted to fat-This means using fat as a source of energy rather than using glucose and getting adapted to this mechanism. Practice intermittent fasting to accomplish it, slightly lower the carb intake, and avoid inflammatory foods.

- Don't Start Too Hard –. Fasting will become easier as your mitochondria become more effective at using fat for food. For beginners, it is recommended to go slow and they can start with the basic form of fasting that is the 16/8 fasting and then they can slowly and gradually shift to other forms of dieting like the warrior diet, etc. Do exercise at the time when you are not fasting and you have consumed enough calories.

Search and eat whole foods. Do Physical exercise. Stay consistent!

Tips and tricks in Intermittent Fasting

1. There should be a reason behind opting for intermittent fasting. It can be about losing weight, improving overall health, or improving metabolic health. The ultimate goal of an individual is to help them determine the most appropriate form of fasting and figure out how many calories and nutrients they need to eat.

2. Indicate clear water when making sure that a good deed can also help clean the system and allow your body to help you do it. Otherwise, to help you with this process, you should evaluate your hiring. The best way to do is to have a glass/bottle of water with you at all times so you can drink.

3. Break in the first place with much luck, the first thing you did after a fast should be a good memory. In addition to the apparent advantages

of healthy food, this also leaves this to eat garbage. Given that you have only 8 hours to eat in your day to day, filling up the supply of good first is always a good option.

4. Respect for the past and your heart. It continues with the certainty that the operation of what needs to do must be sufficient enough to eat every day. The best way to start training should be weight training or every three days. Try to eat most of your diet immediately after your meal.

5. I have never seen the details. One of the real advantages of an intimate fast is that it is not necessary to try to choose other grams of macronutrients. It can be a pain and makes it harder to understand. Follow the rules, and the details will be created by themselves.

Intermittent Fasting Explanatory Guide

Intermittent fasting is the act of not eating for a period of 12 to 24 hours. During this period, you eat nothing and drink only water. Other drinks are also allowed, such as coffee or tea without sugar, but technically this is no longer fast.

Types of intermittent fasting

There are different ways to apply intermittent fasting, and I'm talking about the best known here.

The lean gains method (16h / 8h)

The technique, by Martin Berkhan, was initially developed to optimize muscle gain by doing strength training and practicing intermittent fasting. It is probably the most popular method today, and it is the method that I use and recommend that you test. It consists of fasting for 16h and being able to eat for 8h. For this, it is enough not to eat breakfast.

For example, you finish dinner at 8 p.m., you fast overnight at least noon, nothing prevents you from fasting more if you wish.

The warrior diet

The warrior diet is another method that Ori Hofmekler invented, is older but very close to the Lean gains method. However, no need to define a window of fasting and nutrition. You have to follow your instinct.

The idea is to eat nothing or little in the morning and noon, then have a big meal in the evening. Physical activity during the "fasting" period recommended by Ori. This method is not technically a fast because it allows you to consume some foods in small quantities during the day, e.g., a banana.

The OMAD method (one meal a day) one meal per day

The OMAD method is one of the strictest intermittent fasting methods, the hardest to follow, in my opinion. It consists of taking only one meal a day, a large meal. The objective of this method is to prolong the fasting period in one day as much as possible. If it takes you an hour to eat the big meal, your fasting period lasts 23 hours.

The 5: 2 methods

The 5:2 method developed by Doctor Michael Mosley, and it is mostly thanks to his documentary on fasting "eat, fast, and live for long" that I tested intermittent fasting. The method spread over the week. It breaks down into five days of healthy eating and two days of fasting. On fasting days, you only entitled to a mini-meal of 500 kcal (a large salad).

The Fasti

This method is a French initiative. It's the combination of Thursday and fasting. It was initiated by a French doctor.

It consists of one day of fasting per week, preferably Thursday. You fast 24 hours or more. For example, you no longer eat after dinner on Wednesday until breakfast on Friday morning. It represents a fast of around 36 hours. Or fast yourself until dinner on Thursday for a 24 hour fast. To renew every week.

How to prepare your intermittent fast to make it easier?

Fasting isn't simple, especially in the beginning. However, as with everything throughout everyday life, beneficial things are consistently on the opposite side of the exertion.

Below is a step by step guide to incorporate intermittent fasting in your lifestyle:

First week

You need to do one thing for the initial week. You need to quit breakfast. Why? Two straightforward reasons:

Proceed with the fasting around evening time: each night, we do fasting during our rest. For instance, you quit eating at 9 p.m. at that point the following day you eat at 7 a.m., and you are as of now fasting 10 hours. With no specific exertion. The target of skipping breakfast is to expand this time of fasting from 10h to 16h of fasting. So in our model, if your last supper closes at 9 p.m., you need to include 4 hours to know when you will eat the following day. 9 p.m. + 4 hours = 1 p.m. the next morning.

I might want to call attention to here that nothing keeps you from eating around early afternoon, 11 a.m. or on the other hand a lot later at 2 p.m. if suits you best. You genuinely need to take responsibility for strategy and adjust it to your way of life, and you will build your odds of accomplishment in the long haul.

The other favorable aspect of skipping breakfast is that you will generally use less sugar for the day. The typical breakfast stuffed with sugar. Bread, oat, jam, and milk are sweet and will increase your insulin at the beginning of the day. So proceeding with overnight fasting has a primary extra constructive outcome that will permit you to consume fat and recuperate your digestion.

During this first week, your body will gradually start utilizing your fat as a source of vitality, and it will deliver more ketone bodies increasingly, so your brain functionality remains stable even without eating.

Second week

During this subsequent week, you will proceed not to have breakfast and, additionally, apply two steps, which will help you a great deal to balance out your sugar level for the day and keep it at a moderately low level.

We stop the additional sugars

It is a significant point. On the off chance that you are going to begin intermittent fasting to lose weight is because of your weight, your shape, and additionally, your wellbeing isn't ideal. The additional sugars are, to a great extent, the reason for this circumstance. You need to acknowledge it and counter it.

It is substantially challenging to state that we should stop sugar from being fit. Such vast numbers of beneficial things contain sugar: chocolate, cakes, frozen yogurt. It's practically difficult to maintain distance from sugar. Instead, you need to state that starting now. In the foreseeable future, you will eat the incredibly beneficial things, despite all the trouble—for instance, a birthday cake, extraordinary baked goods that you don't see frequently. The objective is to get the added sugar out of your day by day life. Let's face it, most of the sweet things we devour are not extraordinary, so save this little joy for justified exceptional cases, despite all the trouble.

Indeed, even the sugars, candy and aspartame

During the whole planning time frame and during times of fasting, it is firmly advised not to devour sugars. Regardless of whether they are of the organic source. Here's the reason:

Artificial sweeteners invigorate your body similarly as sugar, at the hormonal level. Your mouth feeling the sweet taste, your pancreas will create insulin so your body can manage your glucose level. A high insulin level obstructs the utilization of fat as a vitality source and subsequently stops your weight reduction. Since you have not expended sugar, your glucose level will drop, and this will cause hunger, best-case scenario, and hypoglycemia in the most pessimistic scenario.

Poor-nutrient starches excluded from lunch
The other point that will assist you with beginning the intermittent fasting is to stop the poor - nutrient starches during the afternoon: bread, pasta, rice, potato, quinoa, wheat, spelled, different seeds, and all that is to flour base. Not exclusively do these foods give you no micro-nutrient nourishment, but they also have the irritating inclination to make your glucose and insulin levels shoot up simultaneously.

The suggested searches are from vegetables, for example, chickpeas, beans, lentils. Sweet potato, squash. These starches give a more significant number of micro-nutrients than the others, contain less sugar, and ingested all the more gradually because they are abundant in fiber.

The objective here is to evacuate dull nourishments that can make your insulin changing a lot after your lunch. It will have the impact of diminishing your hunger and will speed up your utilization of fat as fuel.

Do I have to adopt all of these changes to fast?
Not! These are tips that will help you experience the transition better. If you say to yourself that "I just want to fast and it is out of the question to change my eating habits," then it is not the right time to introduce all these changes, it is not a problem. You can very quickly just fast without changing your habits. Fasting is already a healthy habit that you plan to introduce into your life.

It is better to make a change than to be overwhelmed by all the things we are supposed to do, like eating healthy or playing sports. Once you have adopted fasting and you feel comfortable with it, you can try to introduce a new habit that will improve your health.

How to avoid the inconvenience of fasting?

I will be sincere with you, and fasting is challenging at times. Especially at the start. Hunger tends to decrease over time, but some side effects may appear.

People react differently to a lack of food. We are all different, and the difficulties you will encounter while fasting is probably different from those I experienced.

To avoid the hassles I experienced during fasting, here are some simple solutions, and I think they will help you prevent the inconvenience of fasting.

Cramps

I systematically had foot cramps; at night, when I was fasting at first, it quickly got me drunk. So I took the time to understand the origin of this problem and to test several things to prevent cramps.

An electrolyte imbalance in the muscles causes the cramps. In general, it reflects a lack of magnesium and potassium and sometimes sodium.

I talk very often about insulin in this guide, and this hormone is ultra-important. It also influences our ability to retain electrolytes such as magnesium, potassium, calcium, and sodium. When the insulin level is low, which is the case with fasting, the kidneys retain much fewer minerals. So we end up eliminating much more crystals in our urine than when the insulin is higher. If you start fasting, here's how to avoid cramps:

The solutions

Just take half a teaspoon of pink Himalayan salt every morning. To be diluted in a glass of water. You can also take minerals in the form of capsules during your meals. It strongly advised to supplement magnesium because more than ¾ of the French are deficient, so if you adopt intermittent fasting, you risk worsening this deficiency. High magnesium deficiencies can cause serious problems such as heart rhythm disturbances, so don't take any risks, take your supplements.

The constipation

It is a little embarrassing to approach this subject, but it is essential. Illness can manifest with fasting, it is not systematic, but when it does, it can complicate your task and erode your motivation. Many factors can cause disease in standard times.

Still, if it is triggered only by adopting the fast without any other modification of lifestyle, it signals the same thing as cramps: a lack of minerals.

During fast, overconsumption of water and other drinks is another counterintuitive point that causes constipation. Indeed to fight against hunger, you will probably drink a lot of water, and as explained above, your kidneys do not retain minerals, suddenly you will empty your crystals because you drink too much water. Your body will try to recover as many minerals as possible from your digestive system, and this can lead to constipation.

The solutions
As for cramps, half a teaspoon of pink Himalayan salt every morning. I also advise you to increase your consumption of vegetables, rich in fiber; however, it should not do abruptly, as this can worsen constipation.

Finally, I recommend you to season your dishes well with olive oil or butter, and it helps to lubricate the digestive system properly.

You should drink between 1 and 2 liters of water per day, preferably well spread over the day. You should also drink regularly, highly mineralized waters such as Vichy, St York, and Hepar. If constipation continues, you can take Forex.

Headache

The majority of people who start fasting experience this problem. It is difficult to identify the cause of the headache, but usually, by following the advice below, it will go away quickly.

Before you start fasting, your brain is fueled by sugar. After a few days of fasting, your body will produce ketone bodies. These will largely replace the sugar in your brain. The good news is that ketones are a much cleaner source of energy than sugar.

So be patient during this period of a few days, or your body adapts to your new lifestyle.

The solutions:
If you don't drink a lot, do it! You need to drink at least 1.5-liter water and other herbal teas per day. However, to avoid cramps and constipation, I advise you not to drink more than 2.5 liters.

You also need to consider sleep. The brain is cleaned in the evening, lying down only. So to properly remove the waste from your brain sleeps more than 6 hours, and makes sure you go to bed before midnight.

Hypoglycemia

Hypoglycemia is a sharp drop in the blood sugar level. The average sugar level is between 0.63 gr and 1.1 gr per liter of blood. What you should know is that you can have symptoms of hypoglycemia (weakness, convulsion, unconsciousness) while having normal blood sugar levels. Why?

It happens if you have significant variations over a short period. If, for example, your sugar level, after a meal, goes from 1.5 gr to 0.9 gr quickly, you can have the symptoms of hypoglycemia when your blood sugar is regular—sharp spikes in blood sugar caused by sugars and, to a lesser extent, proteins.

Significant drops in blood sugar caused by high production of insulin. The two are necessarily linked. How to avoid significant variations in blood sugar?

The solutions

The solution is simple and breaks down into two points:

Limit added sugars and carbohydrates low in nutrients such as bread, legs, rice, and potatoes. These carbohydrates don't give you much in terms of nutrients, and they quickly turn into sugar in your blood.

You should know that in our blood, we must at most have the equivalent of a teaspoon of sugar. A bowl of rice contains about ten teaspoons of sugar; inevitably, your blood sugar will increase, and your insulin will also increase, and you will experience a significant variation in blood sugar.

Increase good fats. Indeed fats have a zero glycemic index, so they have no negative impact on blood sugar. So season your vegetables with olive oil, butter. Including fat will generally lower the glycemic index of your meal. What you absolutely should not do is continue to eat large amounts of carbohydrates and increase the number of fat.

Finally, I must remember that you must do your best to eliminate refined sugars from your diet. Refined sugars are the most likely to cause a significant change in your blood sugar.

Deficiencies

It is one of the things that most scares loved ones when someone starts fast. To reassure my wife, I took multi-vitamins for more than a month to assure her that I lacked nothing.

This fear is legitimate, because if during your fast you have a diet low in micronutrients, which is the case in our modern diet, you will probably be deficient. In the short term, the impacts are often invisible because our body will draw on its stocks, but in the long run, it can pose serious health problems.

The solutions

The best solution is also the cheapest is to eat real nutrient-rich foods, especially vegetables. We told every day that we must eat five fruits and vegetables a day. It is the minimum.

Our generation eats less fruit and vegetables than that of our parents, and we are surprised that our health deteriorates visibly.

Fruits and vegetables are very beneficial for our health. They provide us with the majority of the micro-nutrients we need.

To be sure I eat enough, I always take care to build my meals around vegetables. I fill my plate with veggies; I add a portion of protein and sometimes some starchy foods. Another habit that will also allow you not to be deficient in micro-nutrients is to incorporate organ meats into your diet, and I am talking about the liver, heart, kidneys, brain, and kidneys.

These pieces are probably the richest in micronutrients. I must admit that this habit is the most difficult for me to implement. I have never liked the taste of abas since always. Sometimes, when the situation is right, I order offal dishes from restaurants.

A useful cuisine is full of very varied recipes based on organ meats. The best thing to do when it comes to nutrition is to be inspired by these traditional recipes, which highlight these pieces of meats forgotten, unfortunately.

Finally, if the two solutions that I propose to you are not easy to implement in your life. You should take the multi-vitamins of your choice.

Best meals to eat during Intermittent Fasting routine

It is essential to know that the truth is nutrition and find a suitable method that works for you throughout the day. It is the reason why fasting that cannot see is an exciting option when you can change to different approaches. So, an intense and correct diet that compares to another? The answer here is a true reflection. Also, using a 16-hour fast can be a good method. Getting all your thoughts during a good life in almost your entire body of your body goes into action and despairs in body fat. Considered a warm reduction in calories, this is a huge difference. While any reduced calories approach will initially lead to fat-lose, your body is an efficient machine. It will compensate when slowing down metabolism (the exact opposite of what you found) and holding onto body fat.

Is the fasting diet restrictive?

Each diet, by its nature, implies improving with the good ones. If someone is going to sell you with the pancake diet, make a thousand! Trash can never be a good option. However, most people will ask you to start all the time. It is charming to do and directly related to making 12 donuts at once after a couple of ways to find out! An intermittent always also encourages the heart but gives him more room to maneuver. It is difficult to find too much garbage in an unexpected little wind after it has already had its healthy well-being. However, you only need to eat enough to stop everything that happens.

It manifests itself in intimate fasting in various ways and, occasionally, may have had a good selection of one of the best. Each form of intensification of the transformation process had some importance in the panorama that generated success. The best and effectiveness of these distinct differences may differ individually, and it is essential to determine which one is best for you. Also, what may influence which one to choose includes the objectives, which must decide/ routinely, and the current state of life. Most combinations of SE alternate daily on an empty stomach; the diet has been appropriately considered and must be changed.

1. The fasting on alternate days: this always involves alternating days rarely calories of food (or above) with an amount of free food and eat everything you want. It has been shown to help, after the loss and the fat too. Also, it is easier for heart inflammation. The main fall of this intermittent pang lies in the fact that it is the most difficult to consider due to the reaction to hunger during the first days.

2. The modified fasting - diet 5: 2 A proper diet is a protocol with several days of fasting, but then the diet should keep taking some food. Generally, the 20 to 25% of normal always consumed within days; therefore, if you cannot have almost 2000 calories each start day, you could have 400-500 calories for the tastiest meals. Part 5: 2 of this diet suits less strenuous days. In some cases, you can eat almost every five days, so the first or the time remains at 20-25% for two days. This protocol is excellent for weight loss, the composition and also be suitable for regulating the blood, the risk, and inflammation. Studies have shown that the 5: 2 protocols should be as little as possible, improve/reduce the influence throughout the third party (3), and, therefore, show signs of improvements in insulin resistance. In animal studies, this diet has adopted in particular concerning diet 5: 2 taken into account in case of a

reduction of the fat body, in specific hunger (leptin), and in particular for reducing fat bodily. The modified 5: 2 modification protocol can cope with and has had several drawbacks as a result of hunger, but also a bit of irritability at the beginning. Some noticed essential changes, tense tension, and even losing self-confidence and a more positive one.

3. The offer limited in time: if you know that everyone who has said they are doing the right way in which they say, is still in the initial stage of proper nutrition. It is a series of intermittent transfers that have been used daily and are often consumed only during part of the day and do the same for a reason. The ranges of daily fasting in a short time may vary from 12 to 20 hours, more common over 16/8 (the fasting for 16 hours, the user may run 8). For this period, the time of day is not necessary because you keep eating for a consecutive period and

only eat within the allowed time. However, on 8/16, he advised to prepare the meal before the day at 7 in the morning and finished his meal at 15:00 (fast 15:00-19:00) at 9:00 PM or (earlier between 9:00 p.m. and 1:00 p.m.). The protocol does sooner or later, time-to-time, very flexible, depending on what is happening. Timely food is just one of the reasons why we should continue moving forward. The use of this, along with your daily schedule and adjustment, can help you achieve your maximum enjoyment. Limited time research is an excellent weight loss program to improve weight and composition, as well as some other benefits. The new human has meant that weight, reductions in blood flow, and even improvements have been made significantly, even in this case. Some other very positive results from animals have required considering opposing a high degree of insulin, even for the liver. The correct application and the outperformance of a limited period could probably make one great way to lose weight, and chronic thought to begin/start. By mimicking this, it might be better to start, one after another, when it will take around 12/12 hours and finally work up to 16/8 hours.

Intermittent food

Fasting in this segment, let's talk about some foods and the advantages they added in the body in their classes. Let's start with Harissa N.B: before changing the way you eat and altering your diet in any significant way, please speak with a health professional to make sure it's the best decision for you.

HARISSA

Why is it so good for you?

This good pasta or chili still has an excellent and perfect reason. We believe that Harissa may differ, but in general, they always contain a mixture of other ingredients such as peppers, garlic, olive oil, and olive oil. The chile is even more widespread in the world, as is believed to have success and protection against cancer.

How to do it:

It is quite versatile and can be considered not too easy, mixed in others, or stewed, turned into potatoes: the list goes on.

Here is a recipe: all homemade desserts with Black little and Green Harissa.

Nutrition for two tablespoons:

- Calories: 15, Fat: 1 g
- Chloride: 0 mg
- Sodium: 36 mg
- Buy: 2 g
- Unlike fiber: 1 g
- Sugars: 0 g
- Protein: 1 g

GET CHEESE

The reason why it is right for you:
Also, you may feel forgiving, but you got the best of most other cheeses. It also contains the resin, the calcium, and 3% of their daily dose of iron and one-ounce oz. (Some other reason suggests that milk consumption more, the results of milk consumption in strong absorption and

adequate for what we have created.) Is it still not possible? Don't forget that what happened is as good for your health as always.

How to eat it:

However, you like him! It is the reason that others also thought that entries: Quinoa Stuffed Kale GE Rolls with Ches.

Nutrition before 1 hour:

- Claimants: 103
- Passage: 8.5 g
- Chloride: 22 mg
- Sodium: 118 mg
- Carbohydrates: 0.03 g
- Dietary fiber: 1 g
- Sugars: 0.03 g
- Protein: 6 g

POPCORN

Because it is right for you:

Popcorn is a high fiber option that your snack list should include. We are not talking about other popcorn, at least. Compressed air developed without the slightest effort and salty is the best. One suggested that the choice is more satisfying than it is for its irregular shape and its high volume.

How to eat it:

Try to prepare your popcorn on the stove, and it's quick and easy! Apart from the ass, some have thought of someone and a little less.

Nutrition:
- Claimants: 31
- In step: 0.4 g
- Chloride: 0 mg
- Sodium: 1 mg
- Carbohydrates: 6 g
- Unlike fiber: 1 g

- Sugars: 0.07

COCONUT

Why it will acquire for you:

Coconut is an excellent option to create some wealth. It contains potassium, which can help reduce the risk, and some research has also shown that adding some hazelnuts has been useful and makes it fresh too because it is caloric. However, coconut water is not a substitute for real fruit, with some considerations suggesting that the answer does not always meet your nutritional expectations.

How to do it:

Keep the coconut not consumed and dissolved in its jelly and sprinkle on a new juice to prepare a large salad again. With a good wine on top, it's just a good idea, and the small amount of what you add makes nutrients more bioavailable.

Nutrition:

- Claimants: 283,
- After: 27 g,
- Chloride: 0 mg,
- Sodium: 16 mg,
- Candies: 12 g,
- Dietary fiber: 7 g,
- Sugars: 5 g,
- Protein: 2.7 g

ERED-FED MEAT

Because it is good for you:

Much better is lower at all than what can happen in many other types of meat and higher in some fats, as well as omega-3, monounsaturated fat, etc. It's a great source of iron and protein, which is important for growth and development.

How to prepare it:

Whatever you want, prepare yourself as you usually would. Also this way: the grass-fed beef steak starts with sauteed mushrooms

Nutrition for three people:
- Claimants: 99,
- After: 2.3 g,
- Chloride: 47 mg,
- Sodium: 47 mg,
- Carbohydrates: 0 g,
- Dietary fiber: 0 g,
- Sugars: 0 g,
- Protein: 20 g

GHEE

Why is it useful for you?

Ghee is perfect calcium that is obtained by mixing butter and skimming part of the fat. It may be a good idea for someone to say it, and it is the right choice for the persuasions of the Indies. It also has a slightly pleasant taste. It is rich in vitamins and can use as usual for cooking oils or football.

How to do it:

Used as a good alternative for a new flavor and commendable nutritionist.

Nutrition before 1 tablespoon:
- Claimants: 45,
- After: 5 g,
- Cholesterol: 15 mg,
- Sodium: 0 mg,
- LOADED: 0 g,
- Unlike fiber: 0 g,
- Sugars: 0 g,
- Protein: 0 g

CANNED SALMON

Because it is right for you:

Less important than the above, the second version is just one of the best foods with vitamin D that is made for health and absorption of calcium. In its third episode, it is undoubtedly another added advantage.

Come to that:

Canned, sometimes quite small in some, and you will surely want to eat them. They are a great source of calcium that our friends can also create other sources. Frying salmon burgers with toast, as they say, how they eat, and at least, it couldn't be easier.

Nutrition before one year:
- Claimants: 530,
- After: 20 g,
- Cholesterol: 226 mg
- Sodium: 1656 mg,
- Carbohydrates: 0 g,
- Different in fiber: 0 g,
- Sugars: 0 g,
- Protein: 60 g

SPIRULINA

Why it made for you:

Spirulina is a blue-green alga that is less rich in vitamins, nutrients, and antioxidants that make cells grow. It's a good vegetarian source of protein. It can be largely, or in a flabby way, and you are doing your research for a true truth.

How to eat it:

Add a teaspoon of tea to its   more   or   less useful.

Nutrition of 1 spoon:
- Claimants: 20,
- Fat: 0.5 g,
- Chloride: 0 mg,
- Sodium: 73 mg,
- Carbohydrates: 1.7 g,
- Dietary fiber: 0.3 g,
- Sugars: 0.2 g,
- Protein: 4 g

Lemon

Because they made for you:

This fruit can be acidic to create a light orange scent, but it is equally high in vitamin C, which helps to develop blood cells and that healing is important. Not to mention a small lemon, just for each meal, adds a touch of flavor.

How to eat it:

The easiest way of including vitamin C in the diet without taking too is to at least drink once. It is tasty, reassuring, and someone says that if you drink it during the day, it begins to digest during the day. The rest is necessary, but it can't hurt, and it tastes great.

Nutrition for 1 fruit:
- Claimants: 17,
- After: 0.2 g,
- Chloride: 0 mg,
- Sodium: 1 mg,
- Carbohydrates: 5.4 g,
- Unlike fiber: 2 g,
- Sugars: 1.5 g,
- Protein: 0, 6 g.

TOFU

Because you like me:

Tofu is a great example created by someone and is rich in calcium, protein, and iron.

How to eat it:

It is very raw in some cases, and you can do it and do it in a small way to prepare and fry it for an excellent meal. Cover with soy sauce mixed with a little oil, only green, and black pepper and, if desired, a little sriracha.

Nutrition for 1/2 cup:
- Calories: 98,
- After: 5.3 g,
- Chloride: 0 mg,
- Sodium: 15 mg,
- Compact: 3.6 g,
- Dietary fiber: 1 g,
- Sugars: 1 g,
- Protein: 11, 4 g.

DANDELION GREENS

Because they made for you:

The best greens like dandelion are rich in vitamin C and vitamin B, calcium, iron, and potassium. It is an excellent mix for both of us.

How For everything they eat:

In some cases, it has been observed in stock or in this way: pork loin stuffed with dandelion

Nutrition for 1 cup, chopped:
- Colors: 25, Fats: 0.4 g,
- Cholesterol: 0 mg,
- Sodium: 42 mg,
- Carbohydrates: 5 g,
- Dietary fiber: 2 g,
- Sugars: 0.4 g,
- Protein: 1, 5 g.

Purple potatoes

Because they made for you:

I love everything necessary, but the best is rich in potassium - you need to care for the heart. What you're special potatoes are about purple color, which comes from anthocyanin, a powerful antioxidant that poses numerous health benefits like one risk lower for cardiovascular disease.

How to eat it:

However, you would eat a regular potato. Or in this way: Chicken beef and a simple salad.

Nutrition considered as:
- Candidates: 93,
- Fat: 0 g,
- Chloride: 0 mg,
- Sodium: 7 mg,
- Compact: 20 g,
- Unlike fiber: 1 g,
- Sugars: 0 g,

- Protein: 3 g

Real recipes

Why it made for you:

Famous for the crazy good taste (rich in nuts, salty, and somehow supposed) and also for the nutritional punch. Nutrition is also a real recipe with nineteen essential amino acids, such as zinc, selenium, vitamin B, protein, and fiber. (Nutrition is only an inactive part that grew in a field to produce a nutrient dressing).

How to eat it:

Some people call this powerful nutritional propellant "real," but think it is more like a healthy B-vitamin Protein-laced umami boom. It dipped in popcorn with a little life and a little spice. It is also considered as pesto in pesto, or all possible ways, including the fact, or Kale also said so.

Nutrition per ¼ cup:

- Claimants: 60,
- Fat: 0.5 g,
- Chloride: 0 mg,
- Sodium: 25 mg,
- Carbohydrates: 5 g,
- Unlike fiber: 3 g,
- Sugars: 0 g,
- Protein: 8 g

OYSTERS

Because they were for you:

Oysters are a great choice of protein, in addition to 3 acids, iron, calcium, zinc, and vitamin B12. Vitamin B12 is imminent because it keeps the heart necessary and blessed with good health. Indeed, the data on their precedents are as always shorter.

How to do it:

Also, the way someone asked to do something for a great trick was taken by other guests as usual.

Nutrition for 6 media:
- Claimants: 43,
- After: 1.4 g,
- Cholesterol: 34 mg,
- Sodium: 71 mg,
- Buy 2.3 g,
- Different in fiber: 0 g,
- Sugars: 0.5 g,
- Protein: 5 g.

MAGE

Why it made for you:

It is a very versatile fruit, with colors that stand out from gray with a reddish red to bright yellow. Also, they are full of vitamins and antioxidants, particularly for vitamin A: all the rest provides 45% of your daily intake.

Come to that:

Eat it all, in one or more of the 38 best Mango recipes of Cooking Light.

Nutrition for 1 fruit:
- Claimants: 202,
- After: 1.3 g,
- Chloride: 0 mg,
- Sodium: 3 mg,
- Variety: 50.3 g,
- Unlike fiber: 5.4 g,
- Sugars: 46 g,
- Protein: 2, 8 g.

STRAWBERRIES

Because they made for you:

They are a good source of vitamin C and other compounds involved in metabolism and also of them.

How to do it:

No need for our help with this, but here are 20 compelling strawberries created every day.

Nutrition for one year:
- Claimants: 46,
- Fat: 0.43 g,
- Chloride: 0 mg,
- Sodium: 1 mg,
- Candies: 11 g,
- Unlike fiber: 3 g,
- Sugars: 8.1 g,
- Protein: 1 g

BLACKBERRIES

Because they made for you:

Blackberries, in particular, are rich in fiber, which can increase from time to time and satisfied after eating, as are vitamins C, K, and others. The research also linked a good idea of a wide variety of benefits for the body and mind, as the rest helped to take off.

The compounds that produce their colors can also vibrate and also boost the immune system.

Come to eat it:

Bring two of the latter, once again, a couple of glasses of wine and eight cups of milk. Then, turnings out of the fire, leave overnight, and top with blackberries.

Nutrition before 1 cup:
- Claimants: 62,
- After: 0.7 g,
- Cholesterol: 0 mg,
- Sodium: 1 mg,

- Carbohydrates: 14 g,
- Different in fiber: 8 g,
- Sugars: 7 g,
- Protein: 2 g.

ARTICHOKES

Because they made for you:

Some things are much more ecstatic, and herbs are a nutritional potency, a folic acid concentrate, many other fibers, vitamin C, vitamin K and abundant amounts of anhydride, such as quercetin and anthocyanins. When selecting a suitable time to do it, preferably one that is heavy and solid (the weight is less unlikely with a place, as it is).

How to eat it:

It is thought to make some observations, so it is necessary to repeat the outer leaves, peel them. Drink with a simple dip by dipping it in Greek yogurt (or more, if you want a real one) mixed with garlic and curry.

Nutrition for 1 month after:
- Calories: 60,
- Fat: 0.2 g,
- Cholesterol: 0 mg,
- Sodium: 120 mg,
- Compact: 13.5 g,
- Unlike fiber: 7 g,
- Sugars: 1.3 g,
- Protein: 4, 2 g.

SAUERKRAUT

Because it is right for you:

It ferments one-bit fermentation because it contains multiple fibers and fibers that make an excellent addition to the dining table. Something is a good source of iron, manganese, refrigerant, sodium, magnesium, and calcium. No need to mention the fact that it brings a lot of protein to your diet. I like the other perfect way, according to some of the probiotics that adapt to the intestines and digestion.

How to eat it:

You can do the first thing with yourself with the same reason to buy or pre-made and eat it inside, with others, or mixed in others.

Nutrition for 1 CUP:

- Claimants: 27,
- Fat: 0.2 g,
- Chloride: 0 mg,
- Sodium: 939 mg,
- Buy 6.1 g,
- Unlike fiber: 4 g,
- Sugars: 3 g,
- Protein: 1, 3 g.

SPAGHETTI SQUASH

Because it is right for you:

As mentioned earlier, Spaghetti has one of the best waters of all winter squashes. It is often found in many and can be used to replace the substance in many responses. Also, a good dose of vitamin A, calcium, vitamin C, and fiber was obtained.

How to do it:
Turn them into meatballs that you made in the oven.

Nutrition for 1 cup:
- Calories: 42,
- Fat: 0.4 g,
- Chloride: 0 mg,
- Sodium: 28 mg,
- Candies: 10 g,
- Unlike fiber: 2 g,
- Sugars: 4 g,
- Protein: 1 g

APPLES

Because they are right for you:
There are real reflections and a good idea. Apple is rich in a lot of fiber that still may contain cholesterol, transforming them into one way to

start. A little enough to eat apples has allowed people to get at least 15% less than their next meal. One more stupid? They are useful for improving digestion.

How For everything they eat:
Fry a few and then leave with one little honey and apples.

Nutrition from about 1 month:
- Claimants: 95,
- After: 0.3 g,
- Chloride: 0 mg,
- Sodium: 2 mg,
- Candies: 25 g,
- Dietary fiber: 4 g,
- Sugars: 19 g,
- Protein: 0, 5 g.

WILD CAUGHT

Because it is right for you:

The wild cod can be a variety of vitality and sustainability, which is made possible by them. For body fat, fat is in the form of a-3, also called other cardiovascular risks.

How to do it:

Mix a previously created marinade and repeat it in the past.

Nutrition for 3 people:

- Candidates: 71,
- After: 0.2 g,
- Cholesterol: 52 mg,
- Sodium: 114 mg,
- LOADED: 0 g,
- Protein: 17, 4 g.

RHUBARB

Because it is right for you:

It is rich in vitamins and fats, as always.

How to do it:

First, try marinating in rhubarb for a salty kiwi.

Nutrition for 1 tablespoon:

- Claimants: 11,
- After: 0.1 g,
- Chloride: 0 mg,
- Sodium: 2 mg,
- Buy 2.3 g,
- Unlike fiber: 1 g,
- Sugars: 0.6 g,
- Protein: 0, 5 g.

BEET GREENS

Because they are right for you:

It is difficult to understand the correct meaning of beets, but not throw the vegetables that emerge from them. The leaves of some of them, such as paradise and Chiomar vaseline (which have neglected!) Are particularly useful and thought out and can even take into account. They are rich in vitamin A and vitamin K, and one cup contains 44 mg of calcium.

How to do it:
Beet Soup with Potatoes and Grain Beet

Nutrition 1 cup:
- Claimants: 8,
- Fat: 0.05 g,
- Chloride: 0 mg,
- Sodium: 86 mg,
- Carbohydrates: 1.7 g,
- Dietary fiber: 1.4 g,
- Sugars: 0.2 g,
- Protein: 0, 8 g.

PURPLE CAULIFLOWER

Because it is right for you:
As in many cases, the unexpected shade of this cauliflower comes from the old antioxidant. The cauliflower is in many cases and

is fiber, vitamin C, folic acid, vitamin K, and B6 (which always is present in the metabolism and good health). Consider steaming or frying before maintaining high levels of nutrients.

Come to that:

Estimated or retaken at 400° F and then retaken. You need to add oil shine, seeds, and garlic. In the end, add all the other ingredients you prepared, including thyme, mint, and basil. Also, it was considered healthier and purified several times.

Nutrition for 1st comp., Selected:
- Claimants: 27,
- After: 0.3 g,
- Chloride: 0 mg,
- Sodium: 32 mg,
- Compact: 5.3 g,
- Dietary fiber: 2 g,
- Sugars: 2 g,
- Protein: 2, 1 g.

ENDIVE

Because it is right for you:

Endive is rich in inulin and fiber; it can reduce LDL cholesterol levels to improve the situation. Endive is an excellent source of vitamin A and even began as vitamin B, iron, and potassium. Crude often used in some cases, or somehow, it believed that the taste could be pleasant and pleasant.

How to do it:

Drink one little tomato

Nutrition for 1 tablespoon, chopped:
- Claimants: 8,
- After: 0.1 g,
- Cholesterol: 0 mg,
- Sodium: 11 mg,
- As for 1.7 g,
- Dietary fiber: 1.6 g,
- Sugars: 0.1 g,
- Protein: 0, 6 g.

SNAP PEASE

Because they were for you:

Small vegetables are ideal snacks because they are rich in nutrients and fiber and have begun to become raw. A good idea as it might seem more - they are dry, they have a pleasant taste. They are also rich in vitamins A, K, and C.

How to do it:

Peas are delicious dishes or served in hummus, but if you don't want to mix them a little season too, earn some wine or rice vinegar, mix them with some wine, and then.

Nutrition for 1 year:

- Claimants: 31,
- Fat: 0.2 g,
- Chloride: 0 mg,
- Sodium: 6 mg,
- Candies: 7 g,
- Unlike fiber: 3 g,
- Sugars: 3.3 g,
- Protein: 2 g.

CORN

Why it made for you:

An ear of corn has the same value as an apple, with all the levels of nutrients nearly always high. It is not still modified; it is often also loaded with lutein and zeaxanthin, two substances that promote health.

How to eat it:

Roasted Corral in the style of Oaxaca in the CAB

Nutrition for one average year:

- Calories: 99,
- After: 1.5 g,
- Chloride: 0 mg,
- Sodium: 1 mg,
- Candies: 22 g,
- Unlike fiber: 3 g,
- Sugars: 5 g,
- Protein: 4 g

PUMPKIN

Because it is right for you:

It appears to be rich in potassium and magnesium, and pumpkin meat is rich in beta-carotene, which is suitable for the immune system. One of these ingredients contains 7 g of fiber and 3 grams of protein, which is useful for regular digestion. Pumpkin also created 50% of a good dose of vitamin K, which helps prevent adverse reactions.

How to prepare it:

Prepare a cleverly created pumpkin. Throw them in a good dose of basil, olive oil, olive oil, garlic, and yeast. Or again, produced and said as a subsidy or mixed with others.

Nutrition 1 cup puree:
- Calories: 49,
- After: 0.2 g,
- Cholesterol: 0 mg,
- Sodium: 2 mg,

- Candies: 12 g,
- Dietary fiber: 3 g,
- Sugars: 5 g,
- Protein: 1, 8 g.

KIMCHI

Why it made for you:

Kimchi is the source of a good dose of protein and has been used with vitamin A, vitamins B, and vitamin C. Similar to sauerkraut, it also contains its probiotics that need to digest. It gives a touch of flavor to almost all possible.

How to do it:

You can also buy or make yourself. It has a taste appreciated by experts, or you can try it in a recipe like Kimchi Jigae (pork Kimchi-Soup).

Nutrition for 1 cup:

Calories: 22,

After 0, 8 g,

Cholesterol: 0 mg,

Sodium: 747 mg,

Candies: 4 g,

Unlike fiber: 2, 4 g,

Sugars: 1, 6 g,

Protein: 1, 7 g

OLIVES

Why they chose for you:

We know that oil is a perfect ingredient in an extremely delicate way, but we have not found it in its origin. Olive groves are abundant in large part of the fact that this can benefit your heart and your health and maintain weight in any case.

How to do it:

Then, deliver them in some way, or look for them and make them use a recipe.

Nutrition for 1 olive:

- Applicants: 5,
- In the step: 0.5 g,
- Cholesterol: 0 mg,
- Sodium: 32 mg,
- Variety: 0.3 g,
- Dietary fiber: 0.1 g,
- Sugars: 0 g,
- Protein: 0 g.

ASPARAGUS

Because it is right for you:

That said, it is a good source of information, although this is much broader than it is fun, as are vitamins A, C, and K. However, as they say, it also avoids with its recommendations.

Come to that:

Use one another to cut the asparagus into small strips for mixing salads. Also, try them roasted in the oven at 375 ° F for 12 minutes and then put them into practice with the help of a good coffee. There's something very funny about how to make egg yolks with one asparagus.

Nutrition before 1 week:

- Calories: 3,
- Fat: 0 g,
- Chloride: 0 mg,
- Sodium: 0 mg,
- Variety: 0.6 g,
- Unlike fiber: 0.3 g,
- Sugars: 0.3 g,
- Protein: 0, 4 g.

FIGURES

Because they made for you:

This fruit is rich in vitamins C and A and has had a unique way of ensuring that everything is suitable for both sweet and savory. Avoid figs with berries, but they should be a little thicker when choosing what you want to take home.

How to do it:

Try them all tastes like almonds and the cheese to your liking, or make one with these 20 recipes for figs.

Nutrition for 1 fig:

- Calories: 37,
- After: 0.2 g,
- Cholesterol: 0 mg,
- Sodium: 0 mg,
- Carbohydrates: 9.6 g,
- Dietary fiber: 1.4 g,
- Sugars: 8 g,
- Protein: 0, 4 g.

KOHLRABI

Because it is right for you:

This vegetable has a taste similar to that of plants that have an excellent green or purple bulb that often makes the plaster always ready, and you can also leave all its parts. The swede is patina brothers and others and is rich in fiber and potassium.

How to eat it:

They probably stopped remarkably in olive oil or were placed under a chicken so similar to hens. You can also try Honey-Glazed Kohlrabi with Oni and herbs.

Nutrition for 1 cup:

- Claimants: 36,
- Fat: 0.1 g,
- Cholesterol: 0 mg,
- Sodium: 27 mg,
- Compact: 8.4 g,
- Unlike fiber: 5 g,

- Sugars: 4 g,
- Protein: 2 g.

TENDERLOIN PIG

Why it made for you:

The steak vinegar is just created with the American method, such as the heart, indicating that qualifies as said one good meat. Also, it is a large amount of protein, vitamins, and zinc B.

How to eat it:

18 light pork loin recipes

Nutrition from 3 hours:

- Calories: 159,
- After: 5.4 g,
- Chloride: 1 mg,
- Sodium: 55 mg,
- LOADED: 0 g,
- Dietary fiber: 0 g,
- Protein: 26 g.

COFFEE

Why it made for you:

There have been, and then how big is when it comes to the morning cup. But one of every 130,000 after discovering that it cannot increase the increase of health response as disease or cancer, even if you drank 48 ounces. The fact is that, in reality, it is a simple drink, which contains hundreds of different compounds. Some also include oxidants that have associated with a decreased response to type 2, such as Alzheimer's disease, and tells the liver, Romano says.

How to eat it:

Have a good lunch in the morning and drink as much as possible: the advantage is that it was the best, but it is not, and he liked the sugar.

Nutrition 1 cup:
- Calories: 5,
- Fat: 0 g,

- Chloride: 0 mg,
- Sodium: 2 mg,
- Variety: 0.6 g,
- Dietary fiber: 0 g,
- Sugars: 0 g,
- Protein: 0, 7 g.

KOMBUCHA

Why it made for you:

This fermented drink is widespread, as it adapts to the excellent health of the intestine, helps digest, and also takes a nutritious diet.

How to do it:

Kombucha is becoming incredibly fun to be found significant.

Nutrition among the best:
- Claimants: 33,
- After: 0 g,
- Cholesterol: 0 mg,
- Sodium: 10 mg,
- Candies: 7 g,
- Sugars: 2 g,
- Protein: 0 g.

BUCKWHEAT

Because it is right for you:

This whole wheat, which is also Glutin-free, is fiber and is a complete protein. (Curiosity: that's what it takes to make yourself known).

How to eat it:

It can be used as a base for a dish instead of rice, in soups, or tasty as a Belgian buck waffle with waffles.

Nutrition before 1 cup:
- Claimants: 583,
- Fat: 5.8 g,
- Chloride: 0 mg,
- Sodium: 2 mg,
- Carbohydrates: 121.6 g,
- Different in fiber: 17 g,
- Protein: 23 g.

GINGER ROOT

Why it made for you:

The second reason is a natural thing for necessity and movement, as has said and has been used for many years. It not only is spicy but also because it can be better, as does capsaicin, which also has everything to cure and immunize.

How to do it:

If you are worried about having to buy some meat and use only a little, continue in the freezer. Carry it out and let me say that not only because, as has been said, or if you still need one little breathing '.

Nutrition from 5 in total:
- Claimants: 9,
- After: 0.1 g,
- Cholesterol: 0 mg,
- Sodium: 1 mg,
- Candies: 2 g,

- Different in fiber: 0.2 g,
- Sugars: 0.2 g,
- Protein: 0, 2 g.

TAHINI

Because you like me:

Tahini obtained from the soil said that some seeds collected in some cases, for example, also with vitamin E and, therefore, this is also essential, also because it works with B vitamins to help with nerve signaling, average onset, and many contractions.

How to do it:

Tahini is an ideal base for dressings and creams prepared previously. It is also a good dose of Hummus.

Nutrition for 1 tablespoon:
- Claimants: 89,
- Fat: 8 g,
- Chloride: 0 mg,

- Sodium: 17 mg,
- Variety: 3.2 g,
- Unlike fiber: 1.4 g,
- Sugars: 0.1 g,
- Protein: 3 g

BASIL

Why it made for you:

However, this is undoubtedly a member of the mint family, and it is the best of pesto. The other traces of basil also contain an antioxidant that fights inflammation. It is also rich in vitamins, is simple enough to take a good dose of nutrition for many recipes, and is ready with many vegetables.

How to eat it:

You cannot launch it by throwing it first, sooner or later, and continue saying it. The cut or cut has just begun, and it decided to guide the light guide to Basil.

Nutrition for 5 people:
- Applicants: 1,
- Fat: 0.02 g,
- Chloride: 0 mg,
- Sodium: 0 mg,
- Compact: 0.07 g,
- Dietary fiber: 0 g,
- Sugars: 0 g,
- Protein: 0.08 g.

PISTACHIOS

Because they are right for you:

Nelladio, his family life, pistachios are rich in antioxidants, including lutein, but also for pleasure and happiness. They are also rich in vitamin A, essential for vision, and the role of function.

How to do it:

Get along with your brother, and then you can check them regularly and consider them, in this sense, also for broccoli, and then again.

Nutrition per 1 fl oz serving:
- Calories: 159, Fort: 13 g,
- Chloride: 0 mg,
- Sodium: 0 mg,
- Candies: 8 g,
- Dietary fiber: 3 g,
- Sugars: 2.2 g,
- Protein: 6 g.

Spelled

Because it is right for you:

Spelled is beginning to create a good dose of wheat for its nutrients uniquely. It also includes complex and creamy and is rich in solid and excess fiber, vitamin B2, niacin, protein, copper, copper, and copper. He also had fatty and amino acids, which are essential for the fun.

How by E: try this:

Lunch and wild mushroom sauce with pasta.

Nutrition for what you need:
- Claimants: 246,
- After: 2 g,
- Chloride: 0 mg,
- Sodium: mg,
- Buy 51.3 g,
- Unlike fiber: 8 g,
- Protein: 11 g.

SUNFLOWER SEEDS

Why they made for you:

For example, as suggested by the sunflower, for instance, they are rich in vitamin E, which has antioxidant activity that has become fun for immunities. Once soybeans, it has taken fresh from 7, 4 mg of vitamin E, which is 37% of the daily dose.

How to eat it:

Throw them in a portion of some, with oatmeal, or pour a handful sauce and eat them as a path.

Nutrition before 1 hour:
- Calories: 165,
- Fat: 14 g,
- Cholesterol: 0 mg,
- Sodium: 1 mg,
- Candies: 7 g,
- Dietary fiber: 3 g,
- Sugars: 1 g,
- Protein: 5, 5 g.

WATER

Even if you are not eating, you must listen for many reasons, such as how your organ may be from time to time. The amount of anything a person should drink varies, but he wants his urine to be a great color at all times. Dense yellow urine indicates dehydration, which can be useful, stimulating, and light. Combine it with limited foods, and it could be a recipe for others.

If the idea of a meatball has not left you alone, some lemon juice, some remaining mint, or cucumber does it for you. It will be in our best form before. In this case, and also sports drinks because this is also necessary to save energy. Welcoming is a big surprise, since a lot of when you lose sweat during a workout. But after drinking, it is not recommended then, as it immediately cools on your body. Because you have to rebuild the water after a little while completely. You may want to still have a short 'time in the two hours before training and for the reconstruction of those needed to take 250 ml of what had happened during the first or second half by 20-30.

Work out during Intermittent Fasting

It is important to have an understanding that what your body wants before going for exercise during intermittent fasting. Before you initiate any diet or exercise program, consult with your doctor or healthcare provider.

Many experiences benefit women more. At the same time, in four, some experts have faced different problems that can cause incontinence or have already occurred. As for the others, it is necessary to leave the upper part, the harness of more than everything needed to make aging possible. The exercises one can do are sitting, relaxing, or lying, and always involve one firm grip and lift the muscles that float to the muscles differently. A pelvic floor physiotherapist professional once said women should start in a comfortable position and follow the steps below.

Squeeze the muscles around the front of your pelvis, imagine you are stopping urination then squeezing the vaginal walls together pull up through the back passage as if you are stopping wind let go. Do this ten times at maximum capacity without allowing other muscles to help. Once this mastered, a professional said: women should move on to pelvic floor endurance exercise. You do the same task but hold it a little less intense and hold it over a more extended period, the professional says. "It is like going for a jog instead of a sprint."

i. Keep the decision (as detailed above) several times in an appropriate state.
ii. Finish with quick plusses to quickly achieve fusion.
iii. In any case, in this way, at least once such rapid impulses help transform the flow faster for something like sneezing, chewing, and grimacing. If you can do this more frequently and do it at least twice a

day, you will notice amazing results. He added by saying because many might have difficulty finding the right mums and proper correction technique, it can be useful to help you work with a floating pelvis. In any case, the response to these problems manifested with a regular examination that can help improve weakness and also estimate growth. One other way to help an individual to consider these and all these operations will be more after completing the ten assumptions.

JUMP ROPE

It is a perfect Audio movement; it is also an excellent correct movement. It also helps and strengthens muscles, increases fitness, and burns many calories in a small period. Although some see it as a true one, this goes beyond.

QUICK FEET

Also, if your goodwill is the improvement in your mood and good sense, and get a good cardio pulse during the cycle, try to make sure that your feet remain train.

ALPINESTARS

Mountain sports are the right compound exercise and a powerful reinforcement everywhere. The heartbreaking movement shows that your thoughts can still, such as thighs, buttocks, and hips.

BREEDING OF THE SEAT SCHOLARSHIP

It helps in strengthening the inner side, thighs, and calves. One more reason is tears, and even thoughts maintain balance.

REVERSED BOARD

Envying the case is one exercise of enormous scope that strengthens its core, glutes, weight, thighs, and others. If you have decided to put everything in your body for work, it improves stability and flexibility and enhances metabolism.

BASKETBALL SHOT

The fact is that it is a high level, because the whole body improves and adapts, develops strength, and also increases speed and coordination. It is the reason why some aspects, such as the buttocks and shoulders, are the best way to start and begin.

TOUCH AND HOPE

The best way is a cardio-filled movement that challenges your strength and stability and improves durability, courage, and skill. It allowed us to narrow the legs, increase the dose, and lose weight.

Ankle jump

The ankle maintains the tone and carves things, squeezes the heart, and also triggers the aerobic form. This opportunity also increases your skill, coordination, and attention.

CALF HEIGHTS

Cull increases until, as its name indicates, you can. This exercise allows you to increase muscle strength, everything you want to enhance and improve the appearance, definition, and appearance of the latter.

SQUAT BECERRO AGING

The right place for calf rearing is a great exercise to give you the strength of your buttocks and legs. This exercise aimed at the people most affected by others, their calves, but try to maintain a squat.

All these ten exercises will help you if you want your legs to look like high heels; you should also start paying attention to your calves. Stress and goodwill not only seem to escape with a short dress but can also help you increase your athletic commitment and encourage you with a robust solidity. And their decision to exercise on your head, ask your calves, and fight the burning.

Descriptive Recipes For Intermittent Fasting

Information about recipes

These considerations are easy to implement and designed at 5: 2 (2 days in a hurry and five days when you eat rarely) every time you are part of an intermittent diet and, therefore, would do everything possible. These recipes are low-calorie recipes that you can enjoy with your fast, which will leave you full of feeling. All considerations are necessary to start doing so. Adapting the requirements to suit you; all the recipes in this article are different. If you can think of a good part of things, but still it is essential to know how you're eating, so you have to do all the boats to do everything possible.

LIGHTER CREAMY MUSHROOMS IN TOAST

Time Preparation: less than 30 minutes
Cooking time: less than 10 minutes.
For one person

Surely and luxuriously, you will never think that this breakfast is only 200 kcal and counts as one of your five.

NUTRITIONAL VALUE PER PORTION
- Each of them reached 200 kcal
- 17 g of rice
- 14 g of hydrates of carbon (of which 3 g of sugar)
- 8 g before (of which 3 g saturated)
- 3g fiber
- 1.4 g

INGREDIENTS
- One teaspoon of recovered oil
- 80 g / 3 ounces of mushrooms, that's enough

- 32 g / 1 oz of low-fat smoked fats for the first time, just pretty good,
- Two tender onions, thinly sliced
- One tablespoon, also finely chopped
- ½ only small lemon, juiced
- 1 level before starting successfully
- 3 0 g / 1 oz of your choice with olive oil or abundantly prepared
- Season with salt and fry abundantly on the grill to start
- One tablespoon of fresh fruit (first time)

METHOD

1. I took all the oil in a skillet before one another medium. Add the mushrooms, sauce, and onions and garlic and heat for 1-2 minutes. Add the period, and then cover with a lid and look at first a little temperature 'for 5 minutes, or until they have done.
2. Remove from the heat, stir in the batter and thus create, if used, and the season.

3. First, apart from that, place a hot plate and fry the mushrooms.

BANANA MUFFIN

Before the deadline, less than 30 minutes

Cooking-time 10 to 30 minutes

Save six muffins

Ripped added to muffins accordingly, so you don't have to use juice. While flour gives muffins a lot of fiber, it keeps you full at all times.

NUTRITIONAL VALUE PER PORTION
- Each muffin offered 206 kilos,
- 4.5 g of rice,
- 30 g of sugars (of which 13 g of sugars),
- 7.5 g of fat (of which 0.8 g of fat),
- 1 g of fiber and 0.4 seconds

INGREDIENTS
- 125 g / 4½ oz whole wheat flour
- Three light levels should recommend
- 2- standard baking powder
- One half before the start, start
- 50 g / 1¾ approximately for a short time with yogurt

- 50 ml / 2 ml of olive oil, even more, extra for the exception
- Two wavy (175 g / 6 ounces peeled), freshly made

METHOD

1. Before 200 ° C / 180 ° F / 6. Prepare a line of 6-layer muffins with muffins or grease.
2. Mix with the flour, taste, and bake inside out. In a separate bowl, begin to pick up the egg, the egg yolk, and oil. Prepare a well with the flour, add the liquid and mix well. Mix things, as stated, being careful not to mix too much.
3. Pour the mixture into prepared preparations and cook in the oven for 20-30 minutes, or until a response is proposed to make it clean. Also, muffins to a conductive wire can make. Recipe tips: these muffins are frozen, then prepared in batches and frozen for three months.

OMELETTE OF GARLIC MUSHROOMS

Preparation time lasts at least 30 minutes

Cooking-time 10 to 30 minutes

Serving 2

The pleasure and music will bring great excitement to last this to reduce calories, even to make a tortilla. Think also of a simple symmetric and perhaps in a bad mood.

NUTRITIONAL VALUE PER PORTION

As part of an intermittent diet, one before arriving saw 3 of his six averaged every day. It is due to:

- 243 kcal,
- 14 grams of protein,
- 3.5 grams of carbohydrates (of which 3gr of sugars),
- 14 grams of fat (of which 4 grams before),
- 2.5 grams of fiber
- 0.6gr of sale by price.

INGREDIENTS
- Low calorie may be welcome
- Mushrooms 250 g / 9 oz chestnut, sliced
- I left hurriedly, crushed
- One tablespoon chives, sliced
- Four are free, beaten
- freshly ground pepper

FOR THE SALAD
- 1 Little Gem Lettuce leaves the leaves
- 1 00 g / 3 ½ more than what already happened
- 1/3 cucumber, in whole pieces

METHOD
1. Quite a few, flaming frying with oil and placed above a high level. (The reason why it should not be more extensive than about 18 cm / 7 inches). Mix the mushrooms in three batches for 2-3 minutes, or until they are thick and lightly covered. Place the tip in a sieve over a peak to catch all the juices: you

don't want the mushrooms to become soft.

2. Return all oranges and add the herb mushrooms and scallions, and one some green grass abundant. Ask for one more minute, and then you need a way to lose.
3. Remove the grill at its best. Pour the eggs before the months—Cook for five minutes, or at least until instructed.
4. Place the pan under the grill for 3-4 min, or until ready.
5. Compose the salt as an ingredient in a bird.
6. Rediscover the grill and loosen the sides of the restaurant with a long-haired knife. Light a table and continue to do so. I have already seen or said the rest.

CHICKEN BALLS AND VEGETABLES

Before the deadline, less than 30 minutes.

For approximately 30 minutes to 1 hour

Other 2

Try this grilled chicken and balti to get a delicious recipe that is quick and easy to prepare.

NUTRITIONAL VALUE PER PORTION

As already in a secret plan, one portion of approximately 1 in one of its 3 per day after each day 2 of its six days of plant life. This document provides:

- 341 kcal,
- 40 g of protein,
- 30.5 g of carbohydrates (of which 20.5 g of sugars),
- 6 g before (of which 1.5 grams of saturated),
- 9 g of fiber
- 0, 6 g serving previously.

INGREDIENTS
- The calories not sprayed
- One small onion, thin slices
- Four high peaks, created and peeled
- One red prepared studied and released in 3 pieces / 1 piece
- One tablespoon of pepper prepared and cut into three pieces / 1 piece
- 1 tbsp fl corn
- 150 g / 5½z fat-free body fat
- One tablespoon of um or light or strong
- 2, as possible, less has been said
- 227 g / 8 ounces of chopped tin for some
- Three finely prepared with fresh and fresh coriander, other ingredients to decorate finely ground black pepper

METHOD
1. Savor a large, soft pan that does not stick frying pan or with oil and store it in medium heat. Add the onion & cook

for five-min; keep stirring until it is soft and slightly stained.

2. Meanwhile, cut all the possible escape of the thigh legs, but each in four black points and considerate.
3. Add the pasta and other ingredients to the pan with the others and cook for three minutes, turning them immediately.
4. In any case, in a small confusion, mix the pasta with two tablespoons of cold and mix your yogurt until it is thoroughly mixed.
5. Think of the excellent recipe for chicken and vegetables, eat the dish, and cook 30 times.
6. Add the tomatoes to the orange; add the mixed yogurt, 150 ml / 3½ ml of plenty of warm water.
7. Bring and simmer soft for 20-25 min to cook, occasionally
   stirring until the chicken IS tender, and the sauce is thick - season with the

pepper ground freshly black to give the taste and garnish with a carrier.

Crispy Banana and Yogurt

Preparation times: - Pass after 30 minutes.

Time: no need to find

You need: - You need 2

Cream and yogurt are a perfect combination of low calories that will help you spend the night. Goodness had to say it without the need for a first extract, and the seeds bring a satisfying crunch. As part of an intermittent diet.

NUTRITIONAL VALUE PER PORTION

One serving provides its proper dose of fruit 2 of its three every day gradually. It gives 149 partial offers.

INGREDIENTS

- 340 g / 12 ounces before Greek-style natural
- One bath, created and used
- 15 g / ½ oz of mixed seeds (pumpkin, sesame, and Sun) (or used for freshly harvested almonds)

METHOD

1. Divide the yolk between two small birds.
2. Confirm the banana.
3. Sprinkle with some or nuts and serve.

RECOMMENDATIONS FOR RECIPES

Look for mixtures of sunflower seeds, some and sunflower seeds, but it seemed good enough because they are still very high each time.

CAPONATA RATATOUILLE

Preparation time less than 30 minutes.

For approximately 30 minutes to 1 hour

Serves 6

It is rarely a wrapping vegetable that has been able to give rise to the origin of Provence. Perfect for satisfying pleasantly and making people eat too.

NUTRITIONAL VALUE PER PORTION

Your daily style food for 2 of the six virgin daily servings. It provides 90 kilos per serving.

INGREDIENTS

- One tablespoon olive oil
- 750 g / 1 lb 10 ounces of aborigines, in 1 cm pieces
- One large onion, about 1 g / 1½ inches 3 times very thick, chopped enough
- Two large lumps of meat that have chosen, saved and saved
- One chopped time

- ¼-½ teaspoon of pepper
- Two tablespoons capers, drained
- a small handful of fresh cultivated olives
- Four tablespoons white wine
- One spoon of sugar
- 1-2 tablespoons cocoa powder (optional)
- Fresh ground pepper

By genius

Good almonds, carefully and expertly grown

METHOD

1. Keep heating the oil using a nonstick skillet until it is boiling, after leaving the aboriginal and frying for about 15 minutes, or until it is. Add a little 'bombing to avoid doing it if necessary.
2. Once more, put celery and celery into one large pot with a little time '—Cook for 5 minutes or until tender but until firm.
3. Add the tomatoes, leave them, prepare pepper, and start making the pan. Take 15

minutes, stirring occasionally. Add the capers, olives, the wine, cream, and powder and cook for 23 minutes.

4. I have seen one fertile black soil. Divide between 6 roosters, decorate with roasted, thick almonds, and serve.

ITALIAN STYLE MEATBALLS WITH TAGLIATELLE DE ZUCCHINI

Before the deadline, less than 30 minutes.

Waiting time of 10 to 30 minutes

Serves 2

This flat flavorful of Italian meatballs have a healthy twist by using coquette ribbons instead of pasta an easy way to reduce calories.

NUTRITIONAL VALUE PER PORTION

As part of an intermittent plan, one night provides 3 of your six days of vegetables every day. It gives 219 k per portion.

INGREDIENTS FOR MEATBALLS

- 250 g / 9 ounces leaner before (5% fat or less)
- One quite often, very well
- One tablespoon mixed herbs
- you can continue cooking slowly
- One clove of garlic, together
- 227 g / 8 months could change
- Two were created for good after leaving them fresh because they also added

FOR PUMPKINTAGLIATELLE

Two more minutes, trimmed and seeded
Sea and freshly ground black pepper

METHOD

1. Prepare the meat, the other half, with the mixed herbs and a pinch of salt and pepper in a bowl and mix for about ten something.
2. Prepare a medium nonstick skillet with a little oil and cook everything for 5-7 minutes, occasionally turning until golden

brown on all sides. In truth, it was a real success.

3. First, but the rest only in some cases and let simmer for three minutes, stirring. Add the garlic and cook for a few seconds.
4. Mix in this way, 300 ml / 10fl later, the rest mixed and the grated cheese. Bring the bile before starting.
5. Return the other things in the pan, put the stove on low heat and cook for 20 minutes, then stir at least until the sauce is ready, and the meatballs still think.
6. However, fill a half- pot of water halfway with water and bring it to the bile. Use a potato peeler to prepare everything for the tapes.
7. Cook the zucchini in boiling water for a minute and then throw it away.
8. Divide the best strips between two slices and complete them with the sauce and the sauce. Garnish with the left yeast.

CHERMOULA TOFU AND ROASTED VEGETABLES

The waiting time is less than 30 minutes.

Cooking-time 40 min

It serves four people.

By luck, it has also been able to express the flavors of this taste. Serve with freshly cut vegetables for a hearty vegetarian meal.

NUTRITIONAL VALUE PER PORTION

As before an intermittent diet, one night provides 2 of your actual days. This meal includes 182 servings of traditional food.

INGREDIENTS FOR Tofu CHERMOULA

- 25 g / 1 coriander, finely chopped
- Three times he said
- One teaspoon of resin took a little
- 1, we leave the crust finely
- ½ teaspoon dried chili
- One tablespoon olive oil
- 250 g / 9 tons of rice

FOR ROASTED VEGETABLES

- Two someones said, he said
- Two times, said Thickly
- Two red peppers, prepared and chosen
- Two yellow pieces, cooked and sliced
- One small part, according to you
- low-calorie cooking
- already

METHOD

1. Preheat before 200 ° C / 180 ° Fan / Gas 6. For the cream, mix the garlic, the sauce, the lemon zest, and the sauce to add more and a little salt in a routine.
2. Pet a small paper kit and do it in the middle. Cut each half into thin slices. Spread the cream generously over the views.
3. Spread the vegetables in a box of rice and immediately with oil. Continue for approximately 45 minutes, until lightly

stained, turning the ingredients once or twice during cooking.
4. Organize the rest before anything else, with the same extension with the cream, and then cook for another 10-15 min, or until the tofu is light.
5. Divide the plate and vegetables between the four dishes and store them.

YOGUR-BERRY

The waiting time is less than 30 minutes.

Requires unnecessary cooking time

For two persons

Apparently, as a fruitful fruit that is an excellent satisfactory choice, the use of frozen berries makes it a right suspect, they think.

NUTRITIONAL VALUE PER PORTION

As the first of a new diet, one serving provides in your piece of fruit every day two of your three daily meals every day. It offers 149 parts of the price list.

INGREDIENTS

- 175 g / 6 ounces frozen mixed, thawed
- 340 g / 12 feet before Greek cuisine
- 10 g / ¼ of flakes, in my opinion

METHOD

Pour the yolk in two variants, to do it with the best, and then recover the layers. Sprinkle the liquid and spices.

Recipe tips.

You could have left the almonds in a frying pan or bought the lists for the genre.

VEGETABLE SOUP FOR THE HEART

Preparation time less than 30 minutes.
Cooking-time 30 minutes to 1 hour
It serves two people.

This abundant, velvety soup is full of goodness and goodness, perfect to meet on a cold night. If you eat on a short day with an intermittent diet, replace the pieces with unnecessary ones for each day.

NUTRITIONAL VALUE PER PORTION

As part of a different plan, one that serves every time you do it regularly for 3 of your five daily meals. It often reached 219 kcal before the start.

INGREDIENTS

- You can control the cooking or the spray
- One medium onion, see two cloves, thinly sliced
- Two thick, trimmed and thin sticks
- Two medium slices or two peppers, cut into two pieces / 1 in pieces 400 g / 14 ounces canned tomatoes
- One bucket of stock vegetables
- One tablespoon mixed herbs
- 400 g / 14 ounces of tin butter are seasoned and rinsed
- One head of thin plants (approximately 125 g / 4½ ounces), cut and veiled
- said and ground freshly ground pepper

METHOD

1. Spray a large amount of nonstick with oil and see the rest, sauce, sauce, and carrots or peppers gently for 10 minutes, keep stirring until they soften. Add 750 ml / 26 ounces at a time and the other

chopped. Crumble after the fat is gone and mix in the dry flavors.
2. Bring the bile, then recover the form of simmering and wait 20 minutes. Season the soup with salt and soda and add the excellent plums and fillings.
3. Return to a tasty sauce and cook for another 3-4 minutes or until the vegetables soften. I thought about trying and serving in many specialties.

Recipe tips.

Double the risk, if you wish, as an alternative to a choice of people. Others can replace throwing with your other if you don't have one.

LAMB AND FLAGELLET LAMB BEANS

The preparation time is less than 30 minutes

Cooking-time 1 to 2 hours

Serves 4

It was a perfect way to fill your cold. Do not waste time, and this is enough for you to help you comply.

NUTRITIONAL VALUE PER PORTION

As part of an intermittent diet, one serving provides 3 of your six daily meals in your enough daily meal to avoid this is larger than 288 people.

INGREDIENTS

- One teaspoon oil
- 350 g / 12 oz and to the left, according
- 16 crispy onions
- One garlic left, crushed
- 600 ml / 20 ml large broth (produced with a sufficient quantity of food)
- 200 g can choose

- One because you are Garni
- 2 x 400 g can be dried beans, seasoned and rinsed
- 320 g / 11 green ounces
- 250 g / 9 ounces really should
- Fresh and abundant pepper black

METHOD

1. He took the oil in an instant spell or, even later, left the liquor and fried for 3-4 minutes until it was all over.
2. Remove the lamb from the pan and set it aside. Add the first and most often to the pan and fry for 4-5 minutes, or until the onions begin to brown.
3. Return all the pieces in the pan. Add the stock, tomatoes, bouquet garni, and beans.
4. Carry the ball, stir, then before and some time for 1 hour, or until the lamb is only tender.

5. Hurry up, boil a pot of water and blanch the beans. Put in a bowl with ice water.
6. Add the crispy tomatoes to the sauce and season with freshly ground white pepper.
7. Continue shooting for 10 minutes. Divide the stew into four dishes; also set the beans aside and leave them.
8. Recipe tips could be done the night before and then overheated.

CHERRY PACK AND CHERRY FISH

Ready for 1-2 hours

Cooking times of 10 to 30 minutes.

Serve Serves 1

Make the fish is a great way to recover energy. Give the first and the other meat with the chili and cilantro.

NUTRITIONAL VALUE PER PORTION

For this reason, you need one blender or one another plate one once you have found one of his six daily meals available. As part of an intensive diet, 148 people begin.

INGREDIENTS

- 125 g / 4½ oz of steak, little or little steak
- Two tablespoons juice
- One tablespoon first
- One garlic, freshly chopped
- One grated studied and chopped
- ¼ teaspoon of sugar
- Two tablespoons natural yogurt
- 80 g / 3 minutes must think to serve

METHOD

1. Remove the oven at 200° C / 180° Fas / Gays 6. Taste the flavor in a way not too long and stick with the lemon juice.
2. Cover & leave in the refrigerator for 15-20 min. Put the garlic, the garlic, and the red pepper in one good dose of meat and process until the mixture strengthened.
3. Add some sugar, yogurt, and apply the fusion process briefly. Put the meat in a

good dose of the fetus. Make part of both sides with the paste.

4. Collect the tissue without tightening and give the back to seal it. Keep it in the refrigerator for 1 hour.
5. Let stand on a baking sheet and cook for about 15 minutes, or until the dish has prepared—Swabians with scabies.

Pork sautéed with ginger and soy sauce
Timeless preparation in 30 minutes
The waiting time is between 10 and 30 minutes.
For two persons

This little and uncomfortable little pig is fast, and it may be that everything continues to lose flavor and help you have fun.

NUTRITIONAL VALUE PER PORTION
As part of a different plan, one night provides you well enough for 3 of your five daily meals every day, and this is the essential thing for 250 kcal.

INGREDIENTS
- 250 g / 9 ounces for every time everything has been removed but intact
- One tablespoon
- Two tablespoons dark soy
- low-calorie olfactory spray
- 150 g / 5½ ounce buttons, sliced

- Two have been created, thought and chosen
- 75 g / 2½ oz approximately, cut
- 15 g / ½ oz from scratch, but in the meantime very thin
- One garlic left thinly sliced
- Four years before, but in the meantime
- Freshly spotted fresh pepper

METHOD

1. Season the mallet with pepper. Mix the cornmeal with two tablespoons once, until, at least, in some cases.
2. Sprinkle a large pass or remove the frying by cooking and cooking over high heat.
3. Keep stirring the dough for 1-2 min, or until lightly browned, but it has not been possible to do so. Perfect for a dish.
4. Return the heat to the heat, a little heat reset, and start over oil.
5. Sauté the mushrooms and cook for 2 minutes. Add the reseller and leave it for a minute.

6. Then add the ginger, spring onions, garlic, and sauté for a few seconds.
7. Return the kingdom to the person and your place in some way. Continue for 1-2 minutes or until the solution has thickened, and the step has requested.
8. Very immediately.

HOW TO EAT ON QUICK DAYS...?

There is no decision on what or when to start in the next few days. Some probably work better, beginning with a small choice, while others find it better to start as mentioned. However, there are still two million people who have said later: there are other small things often always good, bevel and dinner. Two slightly larger meals: only lunar and dinner. Because the intake is limited to 500 doses of less than 600 calories for men - you are also required to use in your calorie budget. Try to feed on fiber-rich foods that will make you feel full without thinking about too many alternatives. Soups are a good idea for the first days. Studies have shown that they can make it fuller than was said in some original cases or other products with the same caloric content. Here are a few examples of foods that are more adequate days fast:

- An excellent collection of virgins.
- Tasty natural with black cherries
- Purchased or laid eggs
- Grilled with meat or meat
- Cauliflower quarrels
- Some (for example, miso, tomato, cauliflower or vegetables)
- You can choose later
- Black coffee
- Still or how I was playing

Tracking can help you get 5: 2 mass benefits during the one month diet.

Keto and Intermittent Fasting

The intermittent fasting and keto diet are two of the most popular wellness developments of the day.

Many adult men and women use these techniques to lose weight and regularize their guaranteed ailments. Many people wonder if it is entirely free and useful to combine the two.

This article Keto Boost Slim intermittent as well as the keto diet strategy and describes no matter if the combination of the two is a good idea.

What is the Keto Food plan?

The ketogenic diet method (keto) will likely be a superior approach to body fat and decreasing carbohydrate content.

Carbohydrates are often reduced to less than 50 grams per day, which forces the body to rely on fats instead of glucose as its primary source of energy. This diet plan is an excellent technique for losing pounds. When you follow a ketogenic diet program while performing intermittent fasting, it can also provide the following additional positive aspects:

Could speed up your ketosis

Intermittent fasting can help the human body become ketosis much faster than the keto diet program alone. It is the main reason why the body, during fasting, maintains its energy balance by shifting its source of energy from carbohydrates to fats - the basic principle of the prepared keto diet.

By fasting, insulin concentrations and glycogen stores decrease. For those who have trouble in achieving ketosis, during a keto intake system, including intermittent fasting, can eventually and effectively boost up their weight loss.

Do you have to combine them?

Combining the ketogenic diet with intermittent fasting is probably safe for many people. On the other hand, pregnant women and those who have a history of disorderly care should avoid intermittent fasting.

People with specific wellness issues, such as diabetes or heart problems, should seek advice from a health care professional before trying to intermittently fast as part of the strategy.

The bottom line

Combining the intermittent fasting with a keto diet can help you get into ketosis faster than the same old food. It could end up with an overall improvement in the reduction of extra body fat.

However, while this process may work miracles for a few, it is not vital to mix the two, but many people should avoid using this mixture.

You are invited to experiment and find out whether it is a mixture - or only one at a time - that works best for you personally. But as with any critical lifestyle change, it is advisable to speak to your health care provider in an incredibly initial way.

FAQs

Is intermittent fasting dangerous for your health?

In this guide, we talk about intermittent fasting, and it is a fast of fewer than 24 hours. This type of fasting is not dangerous for health and can practice by any healthy person. However, I would like to talk about the following cases where certain precautions must be applied:

People with diabetes: all people with type 1 or 2 diabetes must consult their doctors before embarking on fasting. Fasting naturally induces a drop in blood sugar; combined with medical treatment, the decrease in blood sugar may be too significant. Your doctor should adjust the treatment accordingly.

Undernourished people: people who have a low body mass index, that is to say below 20, should not fast. You should maintain a healthy fat level of your body, neither too high nor too small. It is why being thin is not recommended more than obesity.

Pregnant and lactating women: a pregnant woman needs a lot of nutrients to develop a healthy baby. Many pregnant women are deficient, on specific nutrients, at the start, you should not take the risk of creating additional deficiencies with fasting. It is the same for the nursing woman. It is best not to fast during this time.

Can I drink or eat something during the fasting period?

It all depends on why you are fasting and what type of fasting you are following. This guide is for people who want to lose weight with intermittent fasting.

As part of this goal, I recommend that you eat nothing during the fasting period. As for drinks, you can drink water (still, sparkling), black coffee, tea, and herbal teas. All these drinks must be sugar-free, sweetener-free, and milk-free or vegetable-free—just water to brew your drink.

I read that breakfast is the most important meal, isn't it risky to skip it?
Breakfast, as we know it, is a recent invention. The majority of French people only took coffee with milk and a slice of butter, for simplicity, like breakfast. The breakfast myth has linked to scientific studies showing that people who skip breakfast may experience reduced attention in the morning. If you are not used to fasting, your body at the beginning will run out of sugar because it is dependent on this source of energy. However, once you have fasted, your body produces ketones, which will feed your brain optimally. It will increase your focus and clarity.

The other advantage of skipping breakfast is to eat less added sugar. Indeed at breakfast, the French eat a lot of sugar: cereals, bread, jam, Nutella, chocolate drink, sweet yogurt; in general, breakfast is not a healthy meal at all and brings minimal nutrients.

Can I skip dinner instead of breakfast for intermittent fasting?

Yes, on one condition, have a salty breakfast. The great thing you should know about intermittent fasting is that you can adapt it to your lifestyle. Do you mind skipping dinner less than breakfast? No problem. However, it is essential not to consume added sugar. I say it many times because it is a crucial point. If you skip dinner for a sweet breakfast, your fast may be counterproductive. If you eat at 4 p.m., then you do not eat anything until 7 a.m. the next day, your insulin will go down after these 15 hrs of fasting. A classic sweet breakfast is way too high your insulin.

You are going to cause too much variation in your insulin and your blood sugar level. It will make you hungry quickly.

Are we losing weight?
The answer is yes,"! Thus, studies have shown that alternating fasting (strict) allows you to lose 2.5% of your weight in about three weeks (or almost 2 pounds for a woman weighing 70 kg). Modified fasting, on the other hand, showed that obese people lost 8% of their weight in 8 weeks. It's not huge, but much superior to the low-calorie diet, and you can practice it for as long as you need until you reach the ideal weight and even continue after, once you get used to it.

How much weight will I lose?
The miracle method does not exist. If you fast regularly, you will have results and fast. In the beginning, you will lose a lot, but it is mainly water. Then you will lose slowly.

Depending on your starting weight, the average loss will vary from 250 grams to 2 kg per week, depending on the person. Yes, it is a big range, but we are all different.

What you should not do is conclude after a week of intermittent fasting. For some people, it takes at least two weeks of adaptation so that the body can burn fat quickly and use sugars or fats interchangeably. I, therefore, advise you to test the intermittent youngster for at least three weeks. If you followed the preparation tips above, you would see the results immediately. Otherwise, be patient. If, after three weeks, you don't see any results, you should change your way of fasting. Either you extend the period of fasting, you can extend it up to 22 hours of fasting per day easily. If you haven't, stop adding sugars and nutrient-poor carbohydrates like legs, bread, wheat, and potatoes. You will see the results.

Why is it supposed to be better?

According to several studies, calorie restriction would allow people to live longer in good health. Witness the Japanese supercentenarians who are more adept at frugality than Western-style excess food. By eating less, we put our digestive system to rest, and we "spare" our body (liver, pancreas...).

It also encourages the body to draw on its reserves: it quickly consumes its glucose supply and goes to get its energy from the fats in adipose tissue. Finally, keeping insulin levels low for long periods helps prevent the metabolic disorders involved in diabetes and cardiovascular disease. In a recent study, obese people who followed the 16: 8 fast for twelve weeks consumed an average of 350 calories per day, lost 3% of their original weight, and had their blood pressure drop.

Why can it leave us hungry?

"Beyond a day, I do not recommend fasting in adults because it can upset the mineral balance of the body and increase the risk of tachycardia, renal or heart failure ..." explains Raphael Grumman. The risks of deficiency or fatigue are limited with intermittent fasting, which is nonetheless contraindicated in chronic diseases and people with diabetes. Also, be careful if you take medication morning, noon, and evening, as their proper assimilation depends on regular meals: you should always seek the advice of your doctor.

What if it tempts me?

If you adopt the concept of 16: 8, be sure to balance the other two meals with protein, carbohydrates, and fat. For example, if you skip dinner, don't just eat a "sweet" breakfast. It should contain cheese, a slice of ham, or eggs.

During the fasting period between two meals, continue to hydrate yourself well with water, tea, and everyday herbal teas.

Isn't it restrictive and tiring?

For many overweight people, the method is less painful than a low-calorie diet seven days a week, which is often more frustrating and challenging to maintain. As for the body, it gets used exceptionally quickly, and some people find, on the contrary, they say, a real boost of energy. Usually, once the eating reflex is under control, people find that they are not hungry and rarely suffer from cravings. It is also quite possible to do sports since an experiment conducted on athletes has shown, under intermittent fasting, a decrease in fat mass but the maintenance of muscle mass.

What are the health benefits?

Intermittent fasting methods have shown to have health benefits, and all lead to a rather beneficial increase in basal metabolism (calories burned at rest). In obese people, there is a reduction in triglycerides and blood sugar, an increase in good cholesterol, a slowdown in the heart rate, and a drop in blood pressure. Results demonstrated by medical studies. Even stronger, this alternation of restriction and feast in the mouse showed a decrease in age-related diseases and an increase in life expectancy. It indeed seems to reduce the inflammation of the body and fight against the oxidative stress involved in aging.

Conclusion

It is a famous quote, I don't know who she is, "I've had a lot of problems in my life, and the majority has never happened."

It is useless to ask too many questions. Go ahead! What do you have to lose? If you have any concerns about intermittent fasting, the best way to overcome it or to confirm it is to test it yourself. If you have read negative testimonials about fasting, don't let them demotivate you. Everyone experiences this experience differently. There is no guarantee that cava will match you, but there is a good chance it will shift your health conditions to a better stage.

Made in the USA
Las Vegas, NV
28 August 2021